TRANSFOF
GOES BEYOND

The
3P PROTOCOL

Bio-Hacking Secrets to Quick, Healthy and Sustainable Weight Loss

All the Best! Blessings Dr. F

DR. CHARLES FRANCIS, DC
WENDI FRANCIS MS, RD, CPC

Cover Illustration, Book Design and Production by Efluential Publishing, a division of eFluential Marketing, LLC.

ISBN-13: 978-0-9991949-4-2 Paperback

www.EfluentialPublishing.com

Many thanks to all of the amazing patients that have allowed us to help them throughout the last two decades of our careers. We also want to thank our circle of supportive friends, family, staff and colleagues. Finally, an immense thank you to our children who provide us with enormous light, laughter and love. Without all of you this book would never have been possible.

WHY DID WE WRITE THIS BOOK?

We wrote this book because we have seen so many people really struggle and fail miserably at losing weight and, most importantly, keep it off. Weight loss and sustainable results are truly not hard to achieve if you understand some basic rules of how your body works. This is exactly what you will learn in this book!

Empowering people to lose weight and take control of their body and their life are passions of ours. We know that your weight loss not only affects you but it also, ultimately, affects those that surround you, your children, your spouse, your parents and maybe even your friends. As parents and children ourselves we absolutely understand this and we want to help you change.

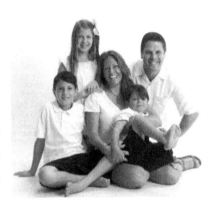

For over 20 years my wife, Wendi, and I have been interested and invested in understanding, integrating and intervening in weight and health change for our patients. Wendi Francis, my wife and co-author of this book, has been working in private practice specializing in all facets of therapeutic nutrition, disordered eating and eating disorders for the last 23 years. Her certifications and trainings have allowed her to save the lives of countless patients, helping them gain weight healthfully if they have had anorexia or lose weight if they were emotionally overeating. More importantly, she also enabled them to change their relationship with food and their psychology of eating, allowing them to ultimately change their life.

Who the Heck are We?

Although I am a Registered and Licensed Dietitian with a graduate degree in counseling and education, my passion for change doesn't stop with the physiology and psychology of our patients. I am passionate about taking change a step further for our clients. As a certified life and business coach, running multiple successful businesses for more 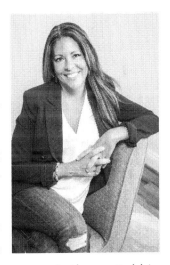 than two decades, and working as an Anthony Robbins Results Coach for a few years, I work to achieve ultimate success in all areas of our client's life. Helping others grow in their health, life and business are innate skills for me and i share my passions in writing, speaking, and private practice. I also work with many professionals and their staff training them in the psychology and physiology of weight and body change, coaching them in specific aspects of their business growth and development. I have completed over 1,000 hours in continuing education and holds certifications in trauma, eating disorders, neurolinguistics programming, grief coaching and life/business coaching.

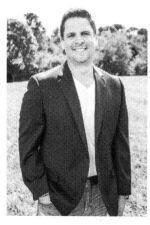

I, myself, have helped countless patients lose weight the healthy way and change their physiology and biomechanics. As I began my career as a Doctor of Chiropractic, I worked with many patients who came to me with chronic back and neck pain, some of which was primarily caused by excessive body weight and having fundamentally inadequate nutrition. I knew that if I did not address the core issue stressing my patients' joints, bones and nervous system, I would never truly enable them to get better. My interest in integrative nutrition grew exponentially as our practice grew. I obtained hundreds of hours of training in integrative nutrition, weight loss and nutrition supplementation. This allowed me to help patients achieve optimal health sustainable weight loss, as well as the health changes regarding disease prevention and treatment.

In our practice, I had a number of professional level athletes and was a TEAM USA Doctor for approximately 7 years. In 2012, I went to London and was invited to the USA house. I worked with all athletes in various 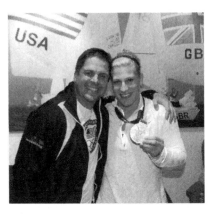 aspects of their health and wellness and loved taking a multi-faceted approach enabling those athletes to achieve optimal results in their physiology and physicality.

Why is This Important?

Because most people who struggle with weight loss have emotional eating patterns that hinder or even halt their short-term success and completely sabotage their long-term success with weight loss. It is important to note that the research shows that 86% of people who have been on more than 2 diets in their lifetime have some facet of emotional overeating.

Weight Loss is Like a Weed

Everyone knows if you only cut the weed at the top and never kill the roots……..the weed is coming back! Simple, right?

Same thing with weight loss! If you or any program you are doing does not address the root issue of emotional eating or medical diagnosis your weight loss success will likely only be short term and keeping the weight off will be extremely difficult or near impossible, which is the real goal anyway! In my opinion this is why so many people (maybe you?) fail at losing weight and usually give up on ever achieving your goals of looking great and being healthy. Why? Because you are only addressing the tops of the weed. How can you expect to be successful?

What are the 3P's?

You see, my wife and I have a passion for helping others change: Change Physically, Change Physiologically and Change Psychologically the (3P'S). Those are the three pieces to success. We absolutely know that without all 3P's, it is quintessentially impossible to change in a sustainable way……that is the bottom line!

Our mission is to treat you as a unique individual, meeting you where you are and providing you with a customized sustainable solution that will allow you to uncover your BEST YOU.

Lose More Weight in Less Time.

Our intention in writing this book is to help you lose more weight in less time, while gaining more physiological health in a sustainable way. That is real success. It pains us both to see any men or women attempt to lose weight by using antiquated methods of weight loss or by focusing only on one facet of weight loss (such as calorie counting or other cookie cutter programs).

This book is here for you to finally put the pieces of your weight loss riddle to rest and to live your life free from weight worries and food issues from this point forward.

Are You Ready?

After all, if you could lose 3 to 7 pounds of fat per week naturally, without exercise, do it consistently, and keep it off.....WHY WOULDN'T YOU? Exactly!!!!

Here is a letter from a patient who may have felt exactly like you before he began our program. At the time he wrote this letter he was approximately 6 weeks into our program.

Dear Dr. Francis and Wendi,
Yesterday I was cleaning up one of my wardrobe armoires and getting it organized. I came across two pairs of designer jeans that I bought at Bergdorf Goodman in two thousand and three after I had suffered life-threatening endocarditis (infected by a dirty catheter during an angiogram) and an aortic valve transplant. I lost a great deal of weight and

many muscles atrophied. There had been an infection in my lower back around the discs and the vertebrae and there was concern they would not heal correctly but thank God they did. However, I was suffering from sciatica even though I had to walk every day in increasing amount of pain.

On one such walk, my, then 13 year old, daughter, Becca took me to Bergdorf for me on Fifth Avenue and took me to what she call the "metro sexual" floor. I accepted this and she prompted me to buy two pairs of designer jeans. By 2006, I was unable to get into those jeans. My daughter was incredibly sweet to me during this time and those two pairs of jeans remind me of how wonderful she was to me when I look at them. Unlike other clothes that have become too small for me, I have never thrown those out.

Yesterday, I pulled them out of the armoire and tried on those jeans. To my incredible astonishment they fit fine. In fact when I was at Eljos later in the day to pick up a repair they commented that they were actually baggy in the butt. Can you believe it?

Thank you. More than 8 inches off my waist. I keep thinking of that ugly yellow fat replica in your office. I have lost at least four of those replicas.

Since 2003, I have faced many health issues. Last Tuesday, I had a visit with my endocrinologist who couldn't stop praising me for having the gumption to do your program. Normally he blasts me for being a smart guy who could not lose weight. All my blood chemistry numbers were normal which hasn't happened in about 35 years, when I was running 6 miles a day in Central Park. I am off my insulin and my blood sugar numbers are fine. The doctor says I will be off several medications probably when I lose the next 20 pounds-November 1, I expect.

I am stunned. I am impressed and I am very pleased.

Thank you.
All the best,
Thatcher S.

TABLE OF CONTENTS

    Why is weight loss so confusing?
    Maybe I should just do surgery, wouldn't that easier?
    Couldn't I just take a pill?
    How is this program different?
    What is the 3P Protocol?
You and Your Food: The Essence of Eating
    Is it true that eating fat makes you fat?
    Do you have fat in this program?
    How can eating fat cause me to burn fat?
    What is the difference between a healthy and a bad fat?
    What is the difference between grass fed or grain fed beef?
    Do I need to reduce my calories to lose weight?
    Is it true eating carbohydrates can make you gain weight?
    What is fiber and what does it do?
    How and why does constipation affect my weight loss?
    How can no calorie foods cause me to gain fat?

How does my thyroid affect my weight?
What is detox and how will it help me lose weight?
Where are these poisons stored in my body?
How can I properly detoxify my body?
Medications
Can my medications cause me to gain weight?
How do my hormones affect my weight loss?
What is cortisol and how does it cause me to gain weight?
Why am I having trouble sleeping?
Why is insulin important if I don't have diabetes?
What is leptin and how does it help me lose weight?
How do I know if I am leptin resistant?

What is a "why?"
I can start a diet but once I "fall off" I can't get back on. What can I do?
What can I do if I don't know how or when to stop eating?
Why is overeating a struggle for me?
What is stomach hunger?
What can I do when I am hungry and when I am full?
What are the other ways to feel hunger?
Emotions and Emotional Eating
What can I do to stop giving in to my cravings?
Why do I overeat?
How can I stop emotionally eating to lose weight?
I am a "sugar addict.' What can I do?
Does stress really affect my weight?
Can the amount of sleep really affect my weight?

I eat at night, sometimes even waking up at night to eat.
What can I do to stop this?
How can I understand my eating and my emotions better?

Introduction

WHY WEIGHT LOSS?
Ignorance is NOT Bliss

What you don't know can kill you and ignorance is not bliss. Here is what we know! Currently, the CDC reports 36 % of US adults are obese which is approximately 73 million Americans. This is still less than the total population of California, Oregon, Washington State, Arizona, Nevada, Idaho, New Mexico all added together.

- It is projected that by 2030 more than 50% of the US will be obese.
- Sadly, obesity affects 17% of our children and adolescents equating to 12.7 million children and adolescents.

Are you in Trouble?

A Harvard study that combined data from more than 50,000 men and over 120,000 women found that:

- Obesity, defined as a BMI > 25, increased the risk of diabetes 20 times.
- Obesity substantially increased the risk of developing high blood pressure, heart disease, stroke and gall stones.

- Furthermore, a review of 15 studies published in the *Archives of General Psychiatry* found that obese people have a 55% higher risk of developing depression.
- High blood pressure is about 6 times more common in people who are obese.

In a study in the *Archives of Internal Medicine* that involved more than 300,000 people found that:

- Being overweight boosted the risk of heart disease by 32%.
- Being obese, BMI greater than 25, increased the risk of heart disease by 81%.
- The Bottom Line in a 2010 study which pooled finding from 19 studies and over 1.5 million people they found that the risk of death increased with body size.

The risk of death from weight related diagnosis ranged from 44% for those were mildly obese, BMI of 30-34.9, to 250% for those with a BMI of 40 to 50.

Did You Know?

- *A 15 pound weight gain doubles your risk for Type 2 Diabetes.*
- *A 22 pound weight gain increases heart attack risk by 75%.*
- *Obesity doubles risk of heart failure and triples risk of Breast Cancer in women.*

(Bradley et. al. The Okinawa Diet Plan. 2004)

Previously, health care providers focused the treatment of obesity on symptoms rather than the cause and prevention. This has not worked. In looking at the statistics, obesity is on the rise for both children and adults. As a country, we are in trouble but more importantly; you as an individual are in trouble!

What is the Better Way?

Integrative weight loss. Policy makers, companies, health insurance industries and corporate wellness programs are all realizing there is a better way to help people lose weight through integrative and preventative approaches.

In this book, we have included the facts that they, and we, know to be true and will change the way you look at your weight loss.

Get the Facts!

Get the facts and get it figured out.

Stop being a statistic: YOU ARE WORTH MORE THAN THAT!

In this book, you will find your most puzzling weight loss questions answered.

Change is quintessentially fear turned outward into action.
--Wendi Francis

PATIENT SUCCESS STORY: MEET BECKI

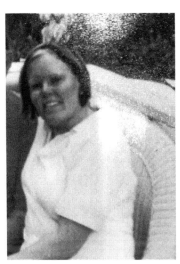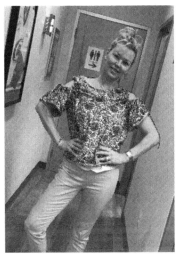

Having been in the medical field for the past 30 years, I spent most of my life caring for others, including my own children and family. Health care workers are "famous" for not taking care of themselves, but we need help like everyone else. I wasn't a food addict or overeater, nor did I have emotional ties to food. I just made bad choices, and didn't take the time to care about my health or myself. After my first grandchild was born, I realized that being in my

early 50's and already having pre-diabetes, high blood pressure, high cholesterol and many other problems required me to take 7 prescriptions a day to control them. I realized that I needed to take control of my weight and my health or I was not going to be around to watch my grandkids grow up. That is when I found Integrative Health Center's weight loss program and got help. With this program I not only lost 52 pounds, but I no longer take any prescriptions on a daily basis, because I no longer have pre-diabetes, high blood pressure, cholesterol problems or any of the other health issues that I had. Nutrition has completely transformed my life and given me my healthy body back. This is something you can't put a price on and something you can't take for granted, but it's something you can achieve with the help of Dr. Francis and the team at Integrative Health Center.

Becki D. ----Health Care Professional

Piece (P) 1
Let's Get Physical

What is necessary to change a person is to change his awareness of himself.
-Abraham Maslow

Why is Weight Loss so Confusing?

It is designed that way for a reason......Profit! Big box weight loss chains and traditional healthcare treatments for weight related illness rely heavily on your business. Not to mention there are a lot of people out there with full time opinions and partial knowledge, which makes them dangerous! Social media is great, however, it has given a voice and platform to everyone, even if they have wrong information or little knowledge.

Here is the Problem:

Most of the time you are taught to only focus on this physical component of weight loss (P1), which is wrong! You might be thinking.....isn't physical change what weight loss is about? Is that why you have tried to lose weight before because you wanted to change the way your body looks and the way your body feels? ANSWER: YES, this is true and NO, it is not really true! Am I confusing you?

The Solution:

If you want true change and sustainable weight loss, then you need to keep reading this book! That is why we wrote this book and what it is all about! You will learn the secrets to weight loss success that the big industries want to keep from you.

So Yes, physical change takes place in weight loss and losing weight takes lots of physical changes, so we will start here by beginning to answer a bundle of your questions to help you in this arena of change and uncovering your best you!

But, know there will be so much more to come in this book.

The number one question we get asked about losing weight is...

Maybe I should just do surgery, wouldn't that be easier?

Many people think this is an easy way to lose weight but in reality, most people don't know the difficulties involved with this surgery. If you think it would just be easier to have surgery because change would be quick and easy, you are wrong! Did you know that you actually need to change your eating habits radically after surgery? And not just a little bit of change, but after bariatric surgery you need to significantly decrease your portion sizes and you may even need to go on a liquid diet for a period of time.

Even before the surgery, the bariatric surgeon will ask you to meet with the nutrition counselor to change your eating and exercise habits. So, in reality you never really get away from changing your food and nutrition. With surgery you will have to be concerned about the multiple complications that can occur, as there is a 1-2% chance of death, and even more possible complications after surgery. These complications include dehydration, malnutrition, lactose intolerance, malabsorption, dumping syndrome, kidney stones and various other issues that can occur throughout the course of the rest of your life.

The majority of Bariatric Physicians, physicians who specialize in weight loss, keep their patients under their care for almost a year pre-surgery, during surgery and post surgery. In this same amount of time or less on our program you could lose an exorbitant amount of weight naturally without all the risks and complications. Not only is it cheaper, but also our program has less risks and leads to a higher quality of life.

Well, couldn't I just take a pill?

Although this trend is decreasing in the United States due to major medical issues associated with approved weight loss drugs, we still wanted you to understand the rationale behind these prescriptions. We are told there are two primary benefits from prescription metabolism booster, also known as catecholamine analogues, such as Phentermine or Benzedrine. First, it will make the hunger go away temporarily, which does not always happen and even if it does it is not a long-term solution. The second possible benefit is that it will possibly lead to an enhanced metabolism. This is supposed to get your body to burn up fat, glycogen and muscle for energy.

The reality is a different story!

A study published in 2001 (and many other studies) showed that when a dieter consumed a higher carbohydrate diet, more insulin, a fat storing hormone, was released. This has a protective effect on the fat cells by overriding the effect of glucagon, your fat burning hormone. This study suggests that the weight loss from these types of pills is actually from burning up muscle and not fat.

The bottom line is if you burn up your muscle, your metabolism will slow down. This is one of the major reasons why you will gain all of the weight back and increase the amount of fat you have on your body. Let's also not forget that your heart is also a muscle.

How is your program different?

In our clinic, we achieve rapid weight loss for our clients in the range of 3 to 7 pounds per week (and up to 1 pound per day) for many consecutive months using a multifaceted approach that targets your Physical, Physiological and Psychological change "The 3P's".

Many patients lose even faster than that in the first month, but I like to give realistic expectations rather than talk about the outliers. If you have struggled to lose four to five pounds per month, it is hard to believe that you could lose up to twelve to twenty-five pounds or more in one month.

What if I am metabolically challenged?

It is important to keep in mind that the majority of our patients are over the age of 40, with many with multiple medical diagnoses, hormone shifts and medications. Many of our clients would be considered metabolically challenged. We often smile when we get to work with someone in their 20's or 30's, because it is easier to accomplish profound change in the health and self-esteem of a young person that will last for the rest of their lives.

Working with individuals who are metabolically challenged may be a little bit more challenging. Despite the challenges, however, we find it to be extremely rewarding because we know we are helping our patients achieve healthy weight loss safely, effectively and efficiently. Many of these patients are also able to reduce or even discontinue some of their medications. We find great satisfaction in knowing we are increasing both the quality and longevity of our patient's lives.

Our 3P's Clinically-Driven, Evidence Based Protocols

In our office we deliver sustainable weight loss and life transformations that go beyond a diet. We identify root causes, eliminate interference, and unlock the full of your potential. Our 3P clinically-driven, evidence based protocols, systematically address the core issues surrounding weight loss and disease prevention.

These 3 P's stand for:

Psychological: focuses on disrupting the link between emotions and eating

Physiological: focuses on changing biochemistry, hormonal shifts and acid/alkaline components

Physical: focuses on weight, contour and nutrient/nutrition change.

We see and enable patients to shed and maintain up to 30 pounds of weight loss in 30 days. Most importantly for us is that we treat the uniqueness of each person with customized, sustainable solutions, uncovering YOUR BEST YOU.

Sounds great, but is it really safe?

Absolutely! I have explained and consulted with multiple physicians regarding our program and outstandingly the consensus is "YES!" Our program was designed with our Clinical Dietitian and we have many medical doctors referring their patients to us for help. Our program uses an individualized, customized approach to weight loss using all natural and whole foods as well as specific supplements to enable patients to achieve their ultimate results naturally, safely and effectively. Our patients not only lose but keep off the weight, allowing their body to change physiologically, from a biochemical, hormonal and metabolic perspective.

You and Your Food: The Essence of Eating

Let food be thy medicine and medicine be thy food.
-- Hippocrates

Is it true that eating fat makes you fat?

No! This is a long-standing fallacy or falsehood. In the early 90's, when we first started in the profession the "fat-free" dieting era was in full swing. As a nation, we saw people's weight increase, nutrient deficiencies increase, early onset arthritis increase and metabolic and hormone issues increase.

You see, eating fat (healthful fat) is critical for weight loss. Fat helps us stay full longer, a concept called satiety. Fat helps us eat less at a meal and can even keep us nutritionally balanced. The only way we can absorb fat-soluble vitamins is by eating fat. If you take fat out of your diet completely you will become malnourished, you will feel hungry all the time, and you will break down your muscle for energy. Essential fatty acids, or fat, can also help with hormone balance, cholesterol moderation, joint health, long-term energy, insulation for vital organs and cell membrane formation.

The problem is that the average American diet contains too much fat and the wrong type of fat. We, as a country, eat too much fat from animal sources. Eating the majority of fat in your diet from plant sources is most beneficial. Read on and I will speak more about this in a few paragraphs.

Do you have fat in the program you designed?

Absolutely but it is from healthful fat sources. Eating fat is essential for health as you can see from the paragraphs above. Without fat in your diet, it is much easier to overeat, become malnourished, and be extremely dissatisfied with your food.

How can eating more fat cause me to burn fat?

Eating healthy fat doesn't make someone fat; it is your body's inability to burn fat that is the real problem. Did you know every cell in your body is comprised of a bi-lipid layer, meaning 2 layers of fat? Fat is not the problem! The answer is understood when you adjust your body from burning sugar, also known as glucose, as your primary fuel to burning fat for you main source of fuel.

What is the difference between a healthy and bad (damaged) fat?

There definitely are healthy fats and unhealthy fats. Typically plant and fish fats are healthier than animal fats because they contain poly- and monounsaturated fatty acids. **Monounsaturated fatty acids** are a type of fat found in a variety of foods and oils. Studies show that eating foods rich in monounsaturated fatty acids improves blood cholesterol levels, which can decrease your risk of heart disease. Research also shows that these fatty acids may benefit insulin levels and blood sugar control, which can be especially helpful if you have type 2 diabetes.

Polyunsaturated fatty acids are a type of fat found mostly in plant-based foods and oils. Evidence shows that eating foods rich in polyunsaturated fatty acids improves blood cholesterol levels, which can decrease your risk of heart disease. These fatty acids may also help decrease your risk of type 2 diabetes.

Many of you may have also heard of **Omega-3 fatty acids.** These are a specific type of polyunsaturated fat that may be especially beneficial to your heart and brain health. Omega-3 fatty acids, found in some types of fatty fish, appears to decrease the risk of coronary artery disease. There are also plant sources of omega-3 fatty acids. Excellent sources of these types of fat include foods such as avocado, coconut, nuts, seeds and various types of oils including coconut oil, avocado oil and olive oil.

Animal fats are saturated sources of essential fatty acids and, when eaten in excess, will cause damage to arteries and create inflammation and disease processes. Hydrogenated oils such as margarine and other animal fats are considered bad fats because of their negative effects on the human body. Hydrogenation is a food processing method. Most fats that have a high percentage of saturated fat or that contain trans fat solid at room temperature, with the exception of coconut oil. Sources of saturated fat and trans fats include beef fat, pork fat, butter, shortening and stick margarine.

What is the big debate about grass-fed or grain fed beef?

Even though beef contains saturated fat there are multiple differences between grass fed and grain fed. Actually, what a cow eats can have a major effect on the nutrient composition of the beef. This is particularly evident when it comes to the fatty acid composition. Grass-fed contains less total fat than grain-fed beef, which means that gram for gram, grass-fed beef contains fewer calories.

The big difference comes in the nutrient composition of the fatty acids. Grass fed beef actually has slightly less saturated fat than grain fed beef.

The biggest difference, however, is that grass fed beef contains up to 5 times the amount of Omega 3 fatty acids and 2 times as much as Conjugated Linoleic Acid, both of these are associated with reduced body fat, better brain and joint health and various other beneficial effects.

Do I need to reduce my calories to lose weight? NOPE!!

According to scientific research, this is a fallacy as well. It is not the amount of calories you eat, it is the source of your food. Many of the people we work with have tried to lose weight by cutting calories and very few have succeeded.

You see it's just not sustainable. You need food and calories, the energy that food provides you to live and help your body work. Calories not only help your internal organs work, (such as your heart, lungs, kidneys and brain), but they also help provide energy for digestion and absorption of nutrients, muscle building, muscle repair, muscle repletion, metabolism, brain function, and many other internal metabolic processes. Without a sustainable caloric intake we cannot function healthfully for a long period of time. This is why most people cannot sustain caloric deficiency for very long.

Anyone who has dieted with severe caloric restriction knows you lose your energy, ability to think, muscle stores and metabolic rate. In a nutshell, it does not feel good and it does not work either!

Is it true eating carbohydrates can make you gain weight?

There are various types of carbohydrate containing foods from sugar/sweet options (please read the section on sugar addiction in the back of this book) to breads and pastas to starchy vegetables all of which contain carbohydrates. All carbohydrates turn into glucose except for fiber. When glucose disperses into your blood, your body automatically secretes the hormone insulin, unless you have Type 1 diabetes and have to give yourself insulin shots.

Insulin helps glucose become glycogen, through a biochemical process, which is then used as energy. Once glycogen stores are full, the extra converted carbohydrates are stored as fat. When eaten in excess all macronutrients, carbohydrates, proteins and fat, are stored as fat. The distinct difference with glucose is its ability to spike insulin. When your insulin spikes in response to a high glycemic food, your fat burning decreases radically, if not stopping altogether. Just understand this, when insulin spikes up, fat burning decreases....it's that simple! Therefore, eating foods with a lower glycemic index and glycemic load can radically reduce the amount of fat stored.

What is fiber and what does it do?

Constipation can exist because of a lack of dietary fiber. Recommended fiber intake for any individual is between 20 and 30 g of fiber per day. In reality, this means eating 8 to 10 servings of whole fruits and vegetables per day. Higher fiber fruits and vegetables include apples, strawberries, raspberries, blueberries, kale, spinach, and broccoli. Remember, without enough fluid (water), fiber will bind more leading to an increase in constipation.

Fiber also helps reduce cholesterol levels as it binds to cholesterol and pulls it out of the body via feces. This enables cholesterol levels to lower and increases your ability to live with less plague in your arteries.

How and why does constipation affect my weight loss?

Going to the bathroom regularly is essential for weight loss as it ensures that your body is moving foods and fluids through and out of it. Bowel movements are a chemical process and your body needs this chemical process to ensure health, metabolic rate and the release of toxins. To help your body have regular bowel movements here are some tips:

- Stimulate peristalsis, the movement of your bowels, naturally. Drink a cup of alkaline water, lemon and Himalayan sea salt every morning upon waking. Heat 8 ounces of alkaline water on the stove until boiling. Pour the hot water into a cup, squeeze the 1/2 of a lemon into the water and put one teaspoon of Himalayan sea salt in and mix until dissolved. Drink it just like a cup of coffee. Do this daily.

- Focus on fiber. Constipation can exist because of a lack of dietary fiber. Remember fiber intake recommendations fall between 20 and 30 g per day. In my experience, the majority of my clients have fallen to less than 50% of this recommendation. Check to see what your fiber intake is first. In our office we use a fiber tracker to help our patients understand this vital aspect of health and weight loss. It is essential in finding out where your fiber intake is before you try to increase it. If your fiber intake is low, increase it to the recommended amounts through consuming more fruits and vegetables. While you do this, make sure your water intake is at least 60 fluid ounces a day to help move the fiber through your body naturally. Know that it can take up three days to see changes in bowel habits.

- Take some magnesium. Magnesium is a mineral that plays an important role in muscle function, heart rhythm, blood pressure, immune system functioning and blood sugar levels. For this reason, magnesium and constipation are directly related, as your entire digestive tract is essentially one muscle. In our clinic, we found that using a natural oral magnesium supplement drink can help alleviate constipation short term. Taking the recommended dosage in 2-4 ounces of water prior to bedtime is most beneficial for constipation relief. Long-term relief from this issue may be found in using a transdermal magnesium cream.

How can no calorie foods cause me to gain fat?

It is not the amount of calories you eat, but the type of food you consume from a nutrient perspective. There are other factors involved such as nonnutritive sweeteners, additives, preservatives, high fructose corn syrup, and other specific sugars that can create an issue with weight gain and toxicity even though your caloric intake is under what your body needs metabolically.

When your body is toxic, it stores these dangerous chemicals in adipose fat (damaged fat) that is found mainly around the chest and belly (spare tire) of men and behind the arms, around the lower tummy, hips and thighs of women. This is part of the metabolic syndrome and weight loss resistance associated with toxicity. Think of fat as storage lockers for toxins. Once the storage lockers are full, your body will add more storage lockers. It is a protective process because it is better to store toxins in the fat than leave then toxins floating freely in your body, potentially affecting your vital organs.

Should I reduce sugar by using non-nutritive sweeteners?

Although the consumption of excess sugar can create lots of different types of diseases, including obesity and type II diabetes, chemical nonnutritive sweeteners are definitively associated with different diseases as well. Various types of cancer, Alzheimer's, dementia and other central nervous system disorders have been associated with specific nonnutritive sweeteners.

However, one of the biggest issues with non-nutritive sweeteners is its relationship with obesity. Diet sodas in particular are associated with an increased risk of obesity. In fact, it has been found through multiple studies that the more diet soda you drink the more likely you are to be overweight. Diet sodas increase sugar/sweet cravings increasing caloric intake far above what you need calorically.

One study of 3,682 individuals examined the long-term relationship between consuming artificially sweetened drinks and weight. The participants were followed for 7-8 years and their weights were monitored. After adjusting for common factors that contribute to weight gain such as dieting, exercising change, or diabetes status, the study showed those who drank artificially sweetened drinks had a 47% higher increase in BMI than those who did not.

"Research shows that sweet taste can increase appetite and the regular consumption of the high intensity sweetness of artificial sweeteners may encourage sugar cravings and dependence," states CNN diet and fitness expert Dr. Melina Jampolis.

The artificial sweeteners in diet sodas also dampen the "reward center" in your brain, which may lead you to indulge in more calorie-rich and sweet-tasting foods, which work against your goals.

In trying to cut sugar intake down, it is most beneficial to use natural alternative sweeteners such as stevia and xylitol to sweeten foods and drinks without sugar.

What foods slow down your metabolism?

Sugar is a major culprit in slow metabolism. Sugar triggers a rapid increase in your blood glucose levels because it quickly finds its way into your bloodstream. This triggers your body to store extra fat and burn fewer calories. Please remember sugar is not listed only as sucrose but also includes high fructose corn syrup, which since the 1960's has become a major additive in various foods and drinks.

High fructose corn syrup is addictive and is one of the major contributors to obesity in our country today.

Dehydration can also radically impact metabolism as water functions in many metabolic processes. Being hydrated is beneficial for your metabolism and your organs as your body can function radically better when it is able to flush toxins and excess waste from your system as well.

One way to cut down on sugar/sweet intake is to use natural foods in a different way to help reduce cravings. In our clinics we use shakes, as well as a variety of supplements, to help clients detoxify their body for 7 days during their weight loss regimen. We use one of the "cleanest" protein powders to help our client's body detoxify and maintain adequate protein status while boosting their nutrition status. Pure Vitality protein powder can be used in a variety of different recipes and calms sweet cravings while increasing nutrient intake for many of our patients as it can be used in some sinfully delicious smoothie recipes.

Here are some examples of these smoothie recipes.

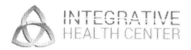

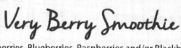

Very Berry Smoothie

(Strawberries, Blueberries, Raspberries and/or Blackberries)

1 scoop Pure Vitality Vanilla Protein Powder
1 cup (8 ounces) unsweetened coconut milk,
unsweetened almond or unsweetened cashew milk
1 cup frozen or fresh berries
(berries with no added sugar, preferably organic)
1 cup ice
Stevia to taste if desired

Put all ingredients into blender container.
Blend on high, until creamy and frothy.

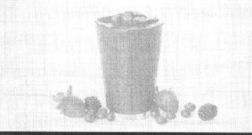

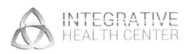

Iced Morning Mocha

6 oz. Decaf Organic Coffee
½ scoop unsweetened cocoa powder
1 scoop Pure Vitality Vanilla Protein Powder
¼ cup Unsweetened Almond Milk
10 drops of liquid French Vanilla Stevia
1 cup of ice

Put all ingredients into blender container.
Blend on high, until creamy and frothy.
Serve immediately

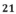

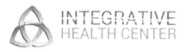

INTEGRATIVE
HEALTH CENTER

Chocolate Raspberry Delight

8 oz. of Unsweetened Almond Milk
1 scoop of Pure Vitality Vanilla Protein Powder
1 tablespoon unsweetened cocoa power
1 cup Fresh or Frozen Raspberries
10 drops liquid Stevia

Put all ingredients into blender container.
Blend on high, until creamy and frothy.
Serve immediately

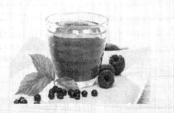

PATIENT SUCCESS STORY: MEET ESTELLE J

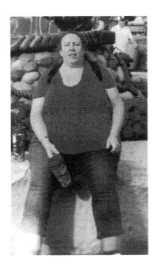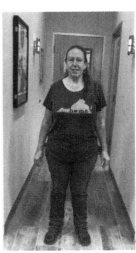

Since I quit smoking almost 30 years ago, I have had a weight problem. At 265 pounds I knew if I did not lose weight I was compromising my health. I watched Dr. Francis' commercials on TV for several months and was skeptical but I made that first appointment. Here I am, 19 months later, healthier, happier and 90 pounds lighter! I lost the 90 pounds in a little over 9 months. Due to a knee injury I was unable to exercise. I followed his plan to the letter. The program is easy to follow, you don't get hungry and the support system is great. I weigh less now than I did over 19 years ago when I married my husband. He is very proud of me.

For years I had borderline high blood pressure. Two weeks on Dr. Francis' program and my blood pressure was normal. My doctor was amazed. Dr. Francis' program works...I am living proof! -- Estelle J

Water, water everywhere...You won't drown drinking water!

The secret of getting ahead is getting started
- Mark Twain

If you lose weight fast, you will gain it back fast. Is that true?

Contrary to popular belief, this is not necessarily true. If you make changes in your food, life and lifestyle, any and all weight loss is reasonable and realistic for the long-term, especially if you get your body into a "fat burning state."

Weight Loss and Fat Loss are Different

When most people lose weight, they are primarily burning muscle weight and not fat weight because they have never shifted their body into a "fat burning state." This is why most people can lose 5-10 pounds on their own (maybe 15-20 pounds) and get stuck. Why? Because your body will not allow you to burn muscle, it is too valuable! Then you get frustrated and go back to your usual patterns and now you gain fat in exchange for the muscle you lost.

Where most people go wrong is thinking that weight loss is only about changing the food you eat. For sustainable weight change, you need to make life and lifestyle change. If you do the physical, physiological and psychological change needed it does not matter how fast you lose the weight. Why, because you are actually burning fat, eliminating toxins and increasing your metabolism. These 3 P's, as we speak about them in our clinic are essential in true and total body transformation.

I hate drinking water! Do I need to drink water to lose weight?

Well, it is essential that you stay hydrated. You can get hydrated from other sources of fluids that do not contain caffeine, such as herbal teas, seltzer waters and juice spritzers. However, these products can be acidic or contain added sugars, which reduces fat burning, so we encourage our patients in our clinic to use them very sparingly and consume the majority of their fluid from pure water.

Alkaline water needs to provide the largest amount of your fluid intake throughout the day. If you do not like plain water try adding lemon, lime or orange slices to it. You can change the type of water bottle or glass you drink from. Many of our clients find that they drink better from different types of containers, whether the water bottles have straws or are large mouthed can make a major difference in how much you drink and how often. I find having water present all day readily available in a container most acceptable to you is extremely helpful. In our clinic we have found that these little things can make the difference between success and failure in this area of wellness. Out of sight is out of mind.

How much water do I need to drink if I want to lose weight?

Research shows and we recommend our patients to consume 1/2 of their body weight in ounces. For example, if you are 200 pounds you should consume 100 ounces of water. That is approximately, only five, 20 ounce water bottles per day! However, please note, that there are certain medical conditions that may dictate specific fluid recommendations different than this. If, in fact, you have a fluid restriction based on a medical condition it is important to stay within those guidelines.

What brands of water do you recommend?

There are many brands of water on the market and it can become very confusing. We always recommend getting water that is filtered or purified.

Filtered water: A countertop or under the sink activated carbon filter is a good choice to remove most chemicals from water.

Better yet, a reverse osmosis filter system will remove even more harmful chemicals in the home. Our own personal units actually filter out chemicals and make our water alkaline as well utilizing a natural process too. No chemicals or electric process to achieve this quality of water that mirrors how water is found in nature.

Bottled water: It is important when choosing bottled water, whether in single serving containers or water dispensing coolers that you check the source of the water and how it is treated.

Some water companies use regular tap water with very little filtration or no filtration. The water industry is not well regulated and stringent purity laws have yet to be established.

In our clinic we advise our patients to drink mineral or filtered spring water, preferably out of glass and not plastic because more and more research points to BPA in plastic causing health problems.

For environmental reasons, we typically suggest that people get a good filtration system in their home and drink bottled water as little as possible to decrease their exposure to BPA, chemical additives and the number of plastic bottles we produce in society. Getting your own filtration unit can save a good deal of money by eliminating water you purchase.

What about alcohol?

In our office, while someone is trying to actively lose weight, we do not recommend alcohol because of its acidity and high sugar content. Alcohol breaks down directly into sugar, spiking blood sugar and triglycerides and hindering weight loss. In fact, drinking alcoholic drinks will actually double the amount of time it takes for you to hit your weight loss goal. Every rule has an exception, and a younger active male may still lose weight even with alcohol. However, if you are 40+ female who has dieted in the past and found it difficult to lose weight, you must stop drinking alcohol in order to lose weight most efficiently.

Another reason we do not recommend alcohol is because the liver metabolizes alcohol. The liver is an integral organ for fat digestion and absorption as it produces bile which is the fluid that helps with fat digestion and absorption. Therefore, alcohol intake can overexert the liver and decrease the body's ability to burn fat.

For some who are social, avoidance of cocktails on a regular basis can be difficult. This is why I have those patients consult with me for an aggressive plan where they double or triple the results compared to the plan I have mentioned in this book.

Is it okay to drink coffee?

Yes, you can have coffee! However, coffee contains caffeine and is highly acidic. It is associated with dehydration and increased acidity. In order to become more alkaline and hydrated we ask people to decrease their intake to 1 cup per day or less. In our clinic we also ask our clients to actually make their tea or coffee with alkaline water to reduce its acidity, ultimately creating more health benefits from an alkalinity standpoint. Being hydrated and alkaline are proven to help with metabolism and have a definitive impact on weight loss.

Patient Success Story: Meet Kathy

WHO LOST OVER 140 IN 11 MONTHS

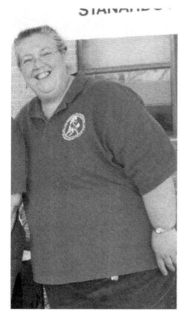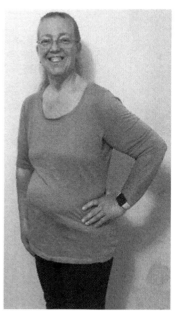

Growing up in an Italian family, the emphasis was always on the joy of looking forward to the next meal. We ate to celebrate life events or to grieve life's challenges. Food was "the constant!"

At a very early age, I knew what I wanted to be when I grew up....A CHEF! So at 12 years old, I worked for a relative in a catering business, took every cooking class available in High School and off to Culinary School I went. After graduation, I worked in many different areas of the food business, got married, moved to Virginia and proceeded to have 3 children. All the while making everyone and everything else the priority over myself. Prior to the program, years before having children, I joined Weight Watchers to help with fertility problems. I was able to lose 55 pounds, but not for long. Three pregnancies in the next 6 years started a weight gain that didn't stop.

Fast forward 20 years, a divorce, elevated blood pressure and knees that hurt ALL THE TIME, something had to change. Meanwhile, I watched my father's health deteriorate due to poor lifestyle. In his 50s', he developed heart disease, diabetes and other chronic ailments. Now, in MY 50's, I decided that was NOT going to be me!

That gave me the impetus to find a program whose emphasis is "real" food for real people. I still cook for a living but have more energy than ever before. I've gone from a size 30/32 to a 12/14 and feel fantastic! I plan on continuing this healthy lifestyle and being a good example to the future generation of my family.

-Kathy B.

Exercise is Not the X Factor

To move is to be alive.--Anonymous

Do I have to exercise to lose weight?

Nope, not at all! In our office, we see many patients who do not desire or are not able to exercise due to physical limitations. This does not hinder their weight loss and, in fact, can sometimes help them lose weight effectively because they are not starting and stopping an exercise regimen.

What types of exercise are best to lose fat?

Burst training is excellent for fat loss. What is burst training? Well, it can burn belly fat fast and involves exercising at 80%–90% of your maximum effort for 20–60 seconds in order to burn your body's stored sugar (glycogen), followed by 20–60 seconds of low impact for recovery. This causes your body to burn fat for the next 24 hours or more to replace your body's vital energy (glycogen) stores.

You only need to do 3–6 sets of 20–60 second bursts 3 times a week to see marked changes and improvements. More is not always better — make sure you have days of rest.

Besides weight loss, are there other reasons to exercise?

1. Boosts brain power by increasing adrenaline, focus and acuity.
2. Decreases stress and cortisol, which decreases fat storage.
3. Increases your energy.
4. Helps with joint health.

Longer is not better!

We now know, the less time and greater intensity is essential for fat and muscle change. Burst or surge training is the way to achieve this.

So what are the benefits to burst or surge training?

It increases muscles stores.

As we age, we tend to rationalize away our ability or inability to exercise. Low to moderate-intensity exercise has been proven to utilize only type I muscle fibers whereas both type I and II muscle fibers are utilized significantly in high-intensity exercise like BURST Training. The loss of muscle mass, often associated with aging, is largely due to the atrophy of Type II muscle fibers which are not worked at all in low-intensity exercise.

It increases immunity.

There is scientific evidence that shows the immune system is suppressed following a cardio or aerobic workout. Plasma glutamine, an essential amino acid necessary for the normal functioning of the immune system, is decreased after long-duration exercise and increased after short-term, high-intensity exercise.

It improves your mood.

Research shows that beta-endorphin levels associated with positive changes in mood state are increased in short-term, high-intensity exercise. This is the opposite of long duration, low intensity exercise. In long duration, low intensity exercise, cortisol is actually released which can leave you feeling good in the moment but can enable you to feel extremely cranky later!

It improves your cardiovascular and respiratory fitness.

Short bouts of exercise (anaerobic) have been shown to produce positive changes in cardiovascular and respiratory fitness when compared to long bouts of exercise (aerobic). Multiple studies show moderate-intensity aerobic training that improved maximal aerobic power did not change anaerobic capacity at all. On the other hand, high-intensity intermittent training may improve both anaerobic and aerobic energy-supplying systems significantly, likely through imposing intensive stimuli on both systems.

It increases HDL cholesterol.

Many people today struggle with varying degrees of cholesterol problems and resign themselves to a life of medication to balance their cholesterol levels. Studies show doing short, intermittent bouts of high-intensity exercise (as compared to slow and steady continuous exercise) increased high-density lipoprotein (HDL) cholesterol levels. This should be very happy news for some of you! Workout LESS and live a longer, healthier life!

Blood pressure regulation.

High intensity exercise is great for many things, and regulating blood pressure is just one more of them! In one study, comparing exercise intensity to exercise duration, exercise intensity had a 13.3 times greater effect on systolic blood pressure and a 2.8 times greater effect on diastolic blood pressure.

Really, how can exercise actually stop fat loss?

As mentioned above, if you are doing long duration aerobic activity (for example, walking 2 plus miles per day), you will be increasing your cortisol levels. Cortisol is a corticosteroid that is released in response to stress and increases abdominal fat storage. For many individuals, this type of exercise increases sugar cravings and fat storage as well as decreasing muscle mass.

Do I need a multivitamin?

In this day and age where most foods contain less nutrients than they used to, it is important that you are get the essential nutrients your body needs. Whether it is through food and/or supplements it is important to maintain adequate nutrient intake status. Liquid or transdermal (cream) vitamin and mineral supplementation is absorbed most effectively and efficiently as it bypasses the gastrointestinal system.

Are there other vitamins or supplements that help weight loss?

Deficiency in specific vitamins and/or minerals can change your body's metabolism, reduce your energy levels, change your mood and alter your body chemistry. In our clinic, we find it essential to use a specific, individualized whole food based supplements to address any and all deficiencies our patients may have, ultimately removing their physiological obstacles to weight loss. In order to ensure our clients had the most effective supplementation, we developed a line of supplements called Pure Vitality. This enables us, as practitioners, to feel safe and certain that our clients are getting an excellent source for supplementation.

Patient Success Story: Meet Phil

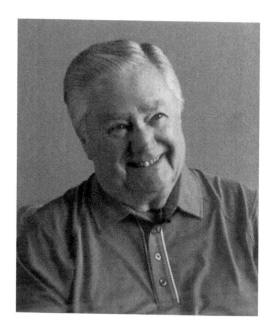

I joined Dr. Francis's diet program with the intent to lose weight. I did not know the benefits that I would realize from the program when I started, I was not only extremely over weight, I had type 2 diabetes and was taking 76 units of insulin every day. I was also suffering from severe joint pain in my knees and had difficulty walking without limping. The pain made it difficult to enjoy playing golf or any activity that required mobility. I contacted my primary care doctor for his input before signing-up since my doctor had experience with another of his patients that had been on Dr. Francis's program and advised me of his success.

Shortly after beginning the program, I began realizing not only did I have weight loss but I was also able to begin reducing my insulin intake and the pain I had been experiencing in my knees was subsiding. I continued losing weight and reducing my insulin intake until I no longer required insulin and my blood sugar was normal. I can now walk normally without pain. I began regular gym visits to maintain my weight and to strengthen my overall body. My Doctor is extremely satisfied with my overall health and my ability to maintain my weight. Thanks to Dr. Francis, and his team, at Integrative Health Center and the health diet. –Phil

PIECE (P) 2-PHYSIOLOGY

There is more wisdom in your body than in your deepest philosophy. -Friedrich Nietzsche

Although focusing on your physical body is important, ultimately focusing on all 3 P's, Physical, Physiological and Psychological, is essential for change and sustainability. This chapter won't be a boring text on your physiology. The physiology of weight loss is about the internal body's ability or inability to change. Knowing how metabolism, toxicity, medications, hormones and alkalinity, play a significant role in weight loss will ultimately empower you to make the essentials change you need for true sustainable weight loss.

Your Metabolism

I heard your metabolism slows down as you age. Is that true?

Metabolism does decrease as you age; however, it is not as drastic as you may think. Between the ages of 20 and 30, your metabolism only decreases 1 to 2% per decade. Beyond that, as you age above 40, your metabolism reduces approximately 3 to 5% per decade. The reason for weight gain as we age is more because of a decrease in physical activity, an increase in toxins, an increase in muscle loss and hormone changes.

Why can't I lose weight now that I am over 40?

Things change as we age, and it's normal. Counting calories is outdated for weight loss, even though this "counting calories" is the foundation for most programs offered today. Everyone has tried the "eat less and exercise more program" and to no avail obesity still exists. To achieve ultimate weight loss success there are specific but simple things you must change in order to lose weight as you age. Things like hormone regulation, thyroid efficiency and muscle depletion, in addition to a variety of other issues to achieve ultimate weight loss success, particularly as you age. Without addressing these things, "the calorie in versus calorie out approach" is doomed to fail.

Abdominal obesity, which is weight gain in the midsection, is one of the telltale signs of hormonal imbalance that we will specifically address in a later question.

It's not that counting calories is completely ineffective. Counting calories may work in your 20's and maybe your early 30's, but it is still a broken method. If you are still looking for a solution to your weight problem after having tried calorie counting please acknowledge there may be more to the problem. The calorie counting theory has other issues when looking at various physiological processes. We will write more on this later.

Will eating after 6 pm make me gain weight?

This is an old fallacy. Eating at specific times of the day cannot make you gain or lose weight. However, if the only time you eat during the day is from 6 pm until bedtime, unless you work the night shift, you will have drastic weight issues because you will have radically thwarted your metabolism. Our body needs to burn the energy from our food consistently throughout the day. When you don't feed your body during the day and then you eat and/or over-eat all evening, weight gain will occur.

If I lose weight fast, will it slow down my metabolism?

No. Losing weight fast does not create a metabolic issue, contrary to popular belief. As long as you make the long-term changes we speak of in this book the weight loss will be long term. Committing to keeping your muscle mass, keeping the changes in your food, and other aspects of your program for quick weight loss will ensure long-term success, in a sustainable fashion.

In our clinic, we have seen many clients lose weight and sustain the weight loss long-term as long as they had all of the "3P's" in place in their program.

How does my thyroid and its function affect my weight?

Your hypothalamus releases TRH (thyrotropin releasing hormone) making your pituitary gland release TSH. TSH then makes the thyroid create T3 and T4 to control your metabolism. When T4 levels are low and TSH is high it is an indicating that your body/brain is trying to force your thyroid gland to produce more T4. This is indicative diagnostically to hypothyroidism. Hypothyroidism has multiple side effects, including weight gain. In our program we address this with a multifaceted approach.

What is a detox and how would it help me lose weight?

Toxicity is an extremely large problem in the United States. Toxins are poisons entering our body through the air we breathe, the food we eat, the water we drink and other chemicals that come in contact with our skin.

There are over 14,000 toxic chemicals the government allows in our food, water, and air, with 75,000 to 80,000 new synthetic substances added to the environment since World War II alone. It is estimated that each person consumes 250 pounds of toxins a year. These poisons in our environment build up in our system causing the body to become toxic.

When the body has had so many destructive toxins put into it for so many years it actually begins to get used to it.

This buildup can lead to many diseases and a variety of painful conditions.

As a toxic load of the body increases, energy levels decrease, and fatigue begins to set in over time. This condition leads to a downward spiral of health where the person will become fatigued, lethargic and overweight.

Where are these poisons that are stored in my body?

They are stored in fat cells. As long as these toxins are in the body, systems that are designed to rid the body of excess fat will not work properly. Losing weight when your body is toxic will not happen easily or efficiently.

How can I properly detoxify my body?

The most important aspect of detoxification is to stop putting toxic food, drink or other chemicals and preservatives into the body. Some toxins in our environment such as food preservatives, air, and water pollution are hard to eliminate. The key here is to do your best and make the best choices you have available.

The second thing to do is eliminate your external or extraneous chemicals such as tobacco and alcohol. After you have a routine established to reduce the amount of toxins you consume, a clean, effective and safe detoxification program can begin as a means of reducing the amount of stored toxins in the body.(Please note that there are many detoxification programs available both online and in stores, so do your research before beginning any program as many are ineffective and/or can be unsafe).

There are many types of detoxification or cleanse programs available. A good detoxification program is one primarily made up of whole organic foods, herbs and nutraceutical support providing a natural and safe detoxification process.

In our office, we personally customize the detoxification program to suit a person's specific need. For most people, we recommend a seven day gentle cleanse with whole foods, herbs, enzymes and supplements that are safe, effective and efficient. This enables your body to release stored toxins in your fat and begin movement with your weight loss.

Detoxification gives your body and your mind a wake-up call that there is something better out there. Once your system is clean it will look and feel better to the extent that it will not want to eat or run on junk food any longer. This allows your body to keep itself clean and toxic free even more, allowing for sustainable health and weight loss.

"A Healthy Outside, Starts from the Inside"
-Robert Urich

MEDICATIONS

Can my medications be causing me to gain weight?

This is a complex topic because some medications will have different side effects in different patients. For example, certain anti-depressants can cause weight gain in some individuals and weight loss in others. This can be perplexing but I wanted to bring you some facts that I know so that you can better judge whether your specific medications may be preventing you from losing weight.

Ironically, some of the medications used to treat obesity related conditions can cause weight gain. Dr. Lawrence Cheskin, Director of Johns Hopkins Medical Weight Management Center said, "Patients and doctors need to be more aware of this, it's an under recognized driver of our obesity problem."

At our office, we create specific weight loss plans for each patient and look at their specific, individual responses to their medications to help them understand how their body is working and whether or not the medications are working for or against them with respect to their weight loss goals. This is one of our biggest secrets to our patient's success. We never recommend a client come off a specific medication, but we do work with their doctors and specialists to decrease or change their medications as necessary and as their health improves. We provide a bridge of support for our clients and their doctors so we can all work together as a multi-faceted treatment team.

Below are just some of the common medications that may cause weight gain. Please do not make any changes to medications you are taking without first consulting with your primary care provider or other specific medical specialist.

Unfortunately, mood and depression can lead to weight gain and some of the antidepressants that are used to treat depression are also linked with weight gain.

Paxil (paroxetine) is one of the big offenders. Serotonin reuptake inhibitors (SSRI's) don't generally cause weight gain. It is believed that serotonin makes you feel happy, satiated and gives you a boost in mood. However, weight gain is commonly seen with patients on Paxil, even though the drug classification as an SSRI is not commonly linked with weight gain.

Prozac is another SSRI that is generally associated with weight loss, but it can have the opposite effect with some people over a longer period of time.

Remeron (Mirtazapine) is another antidepressant that is used to enhance serotonin and norepinephrine, which are related to weight loss. It seems, though, that the antihistamine activity of this drug can increase hunger levels and weight gain.

Zyprexa (olanzapine) or Clozaril (Clozapine) are antipsychotics that increase people's weight as well. A 2005 study found 30% of people on Zyprexa gained 7% more of their body weight within 18 months of taking this drug. (J Clin Psychiatry. 2005 Nov;66(11):1468-76.)

There is another type of anti-depressant medication referred to as Tricyclic Anti-depressants (TCA's). These include Amitriptyline (Elavil and Vanatrip). Tricyclic Antidepressants affect neurotransmitters involved in energy and appetite regulation such as serotonin, dopamine and acetylcholine. But their anti-histamine activity is likely the cause for the weight changes that occur while people are on this medication.

Allergy sufferers who take allergy medications that contain fexofenadine and pseudoephedrine can also gain weight because of the antihistamine action of these drugs.

A 2010 study found that people taking Allegra and Zyrtec were 55% more likely to be overweight than those not taking these medications. (Ratliff JC, *Association of prescription H1 antihistamine use with obesity: results from the National Health and Nutrition Examination Survey.* Obesity (Silver Spring). 2010 Dec;18(12):2398-400.)

This is because the histamine receptor in your body called H-1 acts as an appetite suppressant, and most antihistamine drugs are H-1 histamine blockers. When H–1 is blocked, your appetite-suppressing signal becomes impaired leading to an increase in hunger and eating. While this study didn't specifically identify this as the singular cause of weight gain, the science behind histamine, H–1 blocking, and appetite signaling is a solid correlation.

Diabetes Medications

Individuals who have Type 2 diabetes are typically overweight or obese by diagnosis. If you were prescribed Diabinese (also known as Chlorpropamide),Actos, Glipizide or Prandin (which are sulfonylurea drugs) you will probably gain weight. These sulfonylurea drugs stimulate insulin production, which works to lower blood sugar but may increase your appetite and put your body in fat storage mode.

In our clinical experience, we have documented a number of clients who have not been able to lose weight while on Metformin. As we worked with them to reduce their weight, blood sugars and HGA1C's, their doctors were willing to reduce and/or eliminate their Metformin, which improved weight loss radically.

If you have Type 2 diabetes but also take insulin, you may inadvertently gain weight as well. One study found that people gained nearly 11 pounds on average during their first years of taking insulin about half of that weight gain is thought to occur in the first three months. This puts doctors in an awkward position because without the medication the person's blood sugar would skyrocket but doctors also understand that this starts the vicious cycle of weight gain, which furthers the progression of Type 2 Diabetes.

Correcting this problem requires a very specific protocol where both the doctor and patient work as a team to achieve optimal blood sugar regulation and weight loss at the same time.

Beta-blockers like Tenormin (Atenolol), Lopressor (Metoprolol) or Inderal (Propranolol) can also encourage weight gain.

These medications lower blood pressure by decreasing the heart rate. One study found people taking Tenormin gained approximately five more pounds than the placebo group and research suggests most of the weight is gained in the first few months of using this medication. These drugs can slow calorie burning and create fatigue, decreasing a person's caloric expenditure as well.

Hormones

How do my hormones affect my weight loss?

Hormones can have a significant role in weight gain or weight loss. In speaking specifically about reproductive hormones progesterone, estrogen, and testosterone, there is a significant correlation between an alteration in these hormones and weight gain. Many of our clients have struggled with lowering estrogen levels as they age and increasing abdominal obesity.

Other hormones such as cortisol, insulin and thyroid-stimulating hormone, also known as TSH, play integral roles in weight gain.

The thyroid gland is a tiny gland in your neck that makes free thyroid hormones that increase your metabolism so you can burn up your fat and your energy. A tiny gland in your brain called the hypothalamus and its close relative, the pituitary gland, make a number of other hormones that control the functions of other glands in your body. One hormone made here is your thyroid stimulating hormone or your TSH. This tells your thyroid to start making more free thyroid hormone, which subsequently increases your metabolism. Cortisol stops this hormone from working and will inhibit your metabolism furthering weight gain and abdominal fat storage. I'll speak further on cortisol in the next question.

Insulin, as mentioned previously, is a hormone made by the pancreas that allows your body to use sugar (glucose) from carbohydrates in the food that you eat for energy or to store glucose for future use. Insulin helps keeps your blood sugar level from getting too high (hyperglycemia) or too low (hypoglycemia).

Over 80 million Americans suffer from insulin resistance, which is the body's inability to utilize the insulin it produces which leads to a whole other set of health related problems. Men and women who are insulin resistant have a much greater risk of obesity, diabetes, hypertension (high blood pressure), heart disease, high cholesterol, breast cancer and polycystic ovarian syndrome (PCOS). There is some evidence that insulin resistance may contribute to endometrial cancer. It has also been implicated in Alzheimer's disease.

Insulin resistance is coupled with fatigue and weight gain. As women approach menopause, they become increasingly intolerant of carbohydrates and find it easier to gain weight, especially around their waists. Afternoon blahs, sugar crashes and carbohydrate cravings may all be early insulin resistance symptoms. To lose weight effectively and sustain the weight loss understanding and changing insulin resistance is imperative.

What is cortisol and how does it cause me to gain weight?

I believe cortisol is one of the number one reasons why many people in our country are overweight. Cortisol is a stress hormone, which is secreted throughout the day and is increased during times of stress. Many years ago cortisol was produced to help us move us into "fight or flight" or to go into combat with the saber tooth tiger. Today, we still view threats in the same way and produce cortisol in the same way but do not have the same energy expenditure we once had which allowed us to use the cortisol produced. Cortisol helps break down muscle for energy so you are prepared to run or fight. It decreases libido because reproduction falls to a secondary priority in crisis. It also increases cholesterol and thickens the blood to enable fast clotting in case of injury.

Cortisol has many functions but in general, it helps break things down and tells the body to store fat for time of famine. Remember, stress can be in the form of good stress or bad stress so worrying about bills or throwing a dinner party can be recognized physiologically the same inside the body. In both cases cortisol is secreted and the cascade of events that occurs within the body ensues the same way.

Why am I having trouble sleeping?

When the stress is prolonged, it will start to affect your sleep. One of the jobs cortisol has is to release stored sugar, glycogen, in your liver while you sleep allowing you to maintain brain function. If you overwork your cortisol production glands during the day due to stress they will not be able to produce enough to get you through 8 to 9 hours while you sleep.

Your body, ever clever, will release epinephrine, also known as adrenaline, to break down. When this happens, you wake up in the middle of the night, often times feeling awake and alert due to a burst of adrenaline. Cortisol is needed in the morning to help with the waking process and when this is slow your energy will be low during your morning wake-up routine. Drinking caffeine only makes things worse because you are speeding up a system that is fatigued from running too fast. At this point your body will try to replenish cortisol by creating cravings for ingredients necessary to make that cortisol. These necessary ingredients are things such as fat, sugar and salt. With the additional sweets, fatty, and salty foods your body will now store more fat, particularly around the midsection.

This cascade of events is commonly reported by many of our clients.

This negative cascade effect does not stop there. Cortisol will also inhibit your thyroid hormones. As I spoke about in the question above and as this cascade continues, insulin starts to become involved.

Read on to get more information about insulin-it is just as important about everything else I have spoken of, even if you do not have diabetes.

Why is insulin important if I don't have diabetes?

It is extremely important! Most people think of insulin being a problem for those with diabetes, but insulin is secreted for everyone, any time you eat any food with carbohydrates that contain glucose. Insulin secretions increase when you eat refined carbohydrates such as bread, pasta, desserts, and other sugar oriented foods. It is also released when you eat foods that mix fats and carbohydrates/sugar together such as cheesecake, cookies, pizza, cheeseburger, etc. You get a massive spike in insulin with sugar and refined carbohydrates or fats and refined carbohydrates mixed together. Insulin will drive this broken down energy, in the form of glucose and fat, into the cells so it can be used.

If you have a slow metabolism, fatigue, poor night sleep or an inhibited thyroid, then you must do something with this energy if it is not needed immediately. One of insulin's other jobs is to store this energy as fat so you can use it for another day.

If this cycle of high insulin secretion continues to occur, eventually some of your cells become resistant to insulin. Your pancreas then has to produce even more insulin to get the same response which leads to more weight gain and eventually more insulin resistance.

Insulin will also cause your kidneys to retain more water, which will cause more weight gain from water and can increase your blood pressure as well. This is actually how the cycle of Type 2 diabetes begins.

Long before someone is actually diagnosed with Type 2 diabetes their cells can begin decreasing their response to insulin. This develops into what we clinically say is metabolic syndrome or insulin resistance.

Metabolic syndrome is a condition that is diagnosed when you carry a large amount of fat around your midsection. This typically comes with an increased likelihood of one or more of the following conditions: high blood pressure, elevated blood sugar, high cholesterol, high triglycerides and/or low thyroid function.

In both men and women there is an enzyme called alpha aromatase, which is activated with this metabolic condition. Alpha aromatase converts a female hormone, estrogen, into a male hormone, testosterone, and vice versa in the male.

In women, you will see things like deeper voices, an increase in facial hair and polycystic ovarian syndrome, otherwise known as PCOS, which leads to developing masculine characteristics. Males will develop gynecomastia, male breasts, low sex drive and an increase in body fat stores, among other things. This vicious cycle continues as leptin gets involved as well.

What is leptin and how does it help me lose weight?

Leptin is another hormone your body produces. Leptin has a variety of important functions and one of them is to tell your body that you are full, therefore reducing how much you eat. When leptin stops communicating with your body properly, otherwise known as "leptin resistance", you will continue to eat food and not feel full. Also your body will have a difficult time burning fat, and you will crave carbohydrates and have a difficult time losing weight even with reduced calories and exercise. This leads to more insulin resistance, more bad hormones for men and women, lower thyroid function, and finally, an increase of stress on your body. This also means an increase in cortisol secretion.

Cortisol as you may remember, is the stress related hormone that increases abdominal fat storage.

This cyclical cascade leads further to poor sleep and an increase in cravings for bad food, which further perpetuates this process. This is the vicious cycle you must break in order to succeed with your weight loss.

In our office we reverse this process, break the cycle and reverse the damage with lifestyle, nutrition and dietary changes.

How do I know if I am leptin resistant?

You may be leptin resistant if you struggle to lose weight even with eating less and exercise. You have a high craving for carbohydrates, especially at night and you are storing fat in all the trouble areas. Women tend to store damaged fat, behind the arms, lower tummy, hips and thighs. Men tend to store damaged fat in the chest (barrel chest) and belly (spare tire) but have thin or muscular arms legs.

You may be leptin resistant if you:

1. You struggle to lose weight even with eating less and exercising.
2. You crave high carbohydrate containing foods.
3. You store fat in all the trouble areas. Women tend to store damaged fat behind the arms, lower tummy, hips and thighs. Men tend to store damaged fat in the chest (barrel chest) and belly (spare tire) but have thin or muscular legs.

PATIENT SUCCESS STORY: MEET THE JONES

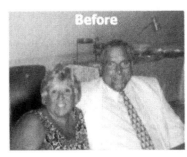
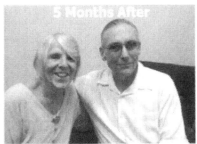

I could not break a plateau of 144 pounds for over 50 years. Every 6 months, I would change to a different diet. I would lose some weight, gain it back again, plus more,50 years of yo-yo dieting. From diet pills, to laxatives, I exercised 5 days a week sometimes twice a day. NEVER getting to 144 pounds. I met with Dr. Francis, I didn't believe him. I decided, "What the hell ...just another diet to add to my hat." Boy! I was in for a surprise, I put down a goal weight of 140 pounds. I blew past it. In 117 days, I was 127 pounds. I has been over 2 YEARS now and I have not gained my weight back. ---C.E. Jones

My weight loss journey has been a life long struggle. I always knew how to lose the weight, my problem was keeping it off. Through Dr. Francis's program I have learned to maintain a constant weight by better understanding of how what you eat effects your body's metabolism, how it stores fats and sugar. I lost 85 pounds on the program and went from 250 pounds to 165 pounds and have maintained a constant body weight between 165 and 170 pounds for the past 2 YEARS. My improved nutrition has been the key. The program works, it is easy to stay with and I am healthier because of it.

-----Jerry A. Jones

Piece (P) 3-The Psychology of Eating

"We know what we are but not what we may be."
Ophelia in Hamlet

Realistically, I know the psychology of weight loss can go in multiple directions. First and foremost, there is the primary facet of psychology that truly embarks on the psychology of change and the mindset needed to change and the psychology behind success and sustainability. This will be the first focus for the number of questions that comprise the beginning of this section.

As Wendi has been an eating disorder and disordered eating specialist for 20 plus years, we would be remiss to not address the questions and issues we tackle and overcome with our patients who have some facet of emotional overeating. Whether diagnostic or not, we know statistically speaking 86% of all individuals who have dieted more than two times consecutively have some facet of emotional overeating. So if you can relate to this, READ ON, as Wendi will cover some specific questions and answers that have radically changed the lives of our patients with emotional eating.

The Psychology of Change- THE 80/20 rule

Success is 80% psychology and 20% mechanics. -Tony Robbins

Let's talk psychology or mindset for a minute. Over the years I have worked with hundreds of clients in my practice, some of which have defied multiple odds stacked against them in getting healthy and/or overcoming emotional or physical insurmountable hurdles. I know, and research supports this, that the psychology of an individual can determine their success or their demise. One of the first distinctions I have been able to make as to why some people succeed and why some people fail lies in their "Why."

What do you mean by Why?

Clients will say "of course I want to get better "or "of course I want to change "or "of course I want to lose weight." Without a distinct and permeating why, long-term sustainable change is difficult. I have learned that in order to be successful you must start with your why.

What is a "Why"?

A 'why' is a particular outcome with which we attach an emotional connection to. So, it's not just, "I want to eat this way because I want to lose weight." That does not change us and it does not connect us emotionally to our outcome.

As human beings if we do not connect to something emotionally we won't continue to strive for success in that area.

It is just a number on the scale but if you get really specific with your 'why' you will be more attached to achieving that number to receive all the things surrounding that number.

- *I want to be able to lose weight so that I can feel stronger in my body.*
- *I can feel more confident.*
- *I can play with my children or my grandchildren and feel playful and joyous.*
- *I can run down the hill after my child is going down the hill.*
- *I can fit better in the seat in my car or a seat in an airplane.*
- *I can shop at any store I want to for my clothes and feel free to be able to purchase things that I love to wear.*
- *I can run down my block and feel strong and powerful.*

You see, in these "why's" there is an emotion with the action. Not just an action. Creating both is extremely important and essential to change and the change parameters. For more information on this topic you can Google Simon Sinek and his TedX talk title "Start with Why."

I can start a diet successfully but once I fall off I can't get back on the diet. What can I do?

As you have set out to embark on the journey of changing your body, there is a key pattern I notice in what I call the backlash of food deprivation that can occur while you are decreasing and changing your food intake. Food deprivation is intense, inexplicable and undeniable. Once someone who is following their diet very strictly eats something off their diet intentionally or not intentionally, all sorts of hell breaks loose in their psyche. In changing anything, but particularly changing your food, your psyche can either be your best friend in the change or your worst enemy against the change.

There is a true psychology to successful eating change. One study reported that for individuals that were told that all sugary snacks were bad, they actually ate 39% more sugar than previously noted. Based on my experience, I would actually say that statistic is radically low. I find the incidence of previously reported rebound binge eating high in our clinic and in the population at large. So how do you get around this? How do you stay forward bound instead of being on the re-bound? There are three things that actually help people in their psychology of eating.

Grey Thinking

First, you must embrace "grey" thinking. People that have black and white thinking or good and bad thinking when it comes to food experience way more guilt/shame, fear and deprivation around their eating or their "not eating." Really, think about it, when someone tells you not to do something how do you respond? If you tell yourself not to do something how do you respond? If you are deprived of something how do you respond? All food is created equal if you allow it to be, by labeling one as "best" and the other as "worst" you create a pattern of despair that cannot be repaired.

In our clinic, our food plan layout is a remedy, a time of healing and repair that the body needs after years of eating poorly. Maybe you have overeaten for a number of years or maybe you have chosen too many of the foods that contribute to weight gain. This plan is a time of your body's reset and recalibration, not necessarily deprivation. As I say to our clients this food is a "not for now food" not a "not for forever food."

The Importance of Your Beliefs

Your belief behind what you are doing is what matters most to the psyche. Instead of saying that you are deprived or on a diet could you say something else? What would that word/words be and how, in converse would that enable you to feel?

Yes, of course some foods have more of this and less of that but the truth is if you look at your foods equally you will actually choose food that your body needs and wants out of an intentional place without fear, guilt, emotion, anger, or anxiety ruling your decisions. If you decide to have that piece of large cheesecake for desert, it is better to have it and enjoy than be tormented by shame, guilt and anger for the next 5 minutes, 5 days or 5 years.

Second, you must understand and accept where you are with your weight, eating and sometimes your emotional patterns before you try to change where you want to go. I often see clients who say I want to lose x amount of pounds or gain x amount of pounds without looking at where they are to begin with or look at the pattern they have displayed in the past with their food or eating. Here is a great example.

Susan was a client of ours who wanted to lose 70 pounds. All she could talk about was how much she hated herself, her eating and her weight. She was afraid to fail and did not want to write down what she had been eating. She was also just as afraid to begin a new way of eating. In a session with me, she saw that she was using her emotions as an obstacle to her change. In admitting, understanding, accepting and changing her shame/guilt cycle she began to rid herself of the negative emotions associated with her weight and her food. Then, and only then, could she accept where she was and begin to change the cycle and patterns, not just emotionally but physically and physiologically as well, leading to radical success for her weight loss.

You see, you cannot change yourself until you understand and accept where you are. To get back up and begin to change again you must understand and accept where you are to determine if where you want to go is appropriate for you, it is realistic and achievable? If not you must make it realistic, objective and emotionally sound in order to get up and start the change that leads to sustainable weight loss.

Belief = Behavior

Thirdly, do not overlook your thoughts and beliefs about food. Thoughts plus beliefs equals behavior. You cannot change any behavior in a way that lasts unless you change your thoughts and beliefs around that change. If you don't believe you can be a certain weight or size or eat a certain way, you need to start by changing your belief as you change your behavior. We do not change from the outside in when it comes to food change; we change from the inside out. Get clear on what your beliefs and thoughts are and begin to change those in order to achieve true, sustainable success.

Falling off the Wagon

Specifically when you "fall off the wagon" by eating something not on your plan there are a few things you can do to get back up

1. Brush it off. Shame, blame and guilt do not work. Negative focus leads to negative feelings, which leads to negative actions. This is NOT a free pass to keep eating or to berate yourself. Don't use your food against you. Overeating or eating off your plan

is a behavior. Your behavior is what you do, NOT who you are.

2. Learn from it objectively. What can it teach you about your pattern/patterns? Could it be you got too hungry? Could it be you were in a deprivation related pattern? See the mistake from a bird's eye perspective.

3. Move on and reconfigure. Focus on the solutions instead of the problem. Ask questions like what can I do different next time? What prevented me from doing what I knew I needed to do?

4. Focus on what you have done right for that day and start again. None of us learned to walk by falling down the first time and staying on the ground.

Part of my issue is that I do not feel fullness anymore. What can I do if I don't know how or when to stop eating?

On Hunger and Fullness....

> *Practice isn't' the things you do once you are good, it's the thing you do that makes you good.*
> *-Malcom Gladwell*

For years, I have worked with clients struggling with hunger and fullness patterns. So often I have heard things like:

"I don't know when I am full so I can't stop."

"It just tastes so good, I can't stop eating it!"

"I never let myself get hungry, I am afraid that if I get too hungry I will start eating and not stop!"

Hunger and fullness are signals that the hypothalamus in the brain controls to tell the body when to stop and start eating. We are all born with the ability to have this happen internally with no external cues. However, things can go awry with this and in my experience in three very distinct areas of life:

1. **Early childhood:** If caregivers feed in response to emotions like using food as comfort or for calming anxiety, or potentially if they take away food in response to emotions like using food as a reward system or using food as threat hunger signals can go awry. This is because feeding is based on emotional input or external regulation parameters, like the "clean your plate club."

2. **Adolescence:** When emotions are running higher and brain changes in the reward system area are locked, as is the case in adolescence, learning connection with food in loneliness or happiness on a regular basis can lead to significant emotional connections with food.

   "When I was a teenager, I was socially awkward so I liked to get a good book and eat all night-that was my one escape from my life" -client quote.

   Also, radical difference between adolescent eating and adult eating is important to note as adolescents need to eat on a different schedule than adults because of their specific hormonal and energy expenditure patterns. When you make adolescents eat on an "adult schedule" you teach them to override their internal hunger and fullness patterns.

3. **Adulthood.** If you have been on multiple diets, you have learned to override your hunger and fullness signals for many months or potentially many years. You may also override fullness signals as you begin eating again after a diet in order to feel satiated emotionally from the deprivation that ensued.

Eating when you're hungry and stopping when you're full sounds simple yet, countless people, struggle with understanding and putting this principle into practice.

Why is over eating such a struggle for me?

You are not alone. There are many people out there just like you. One of the main reasons overeating is a problem is because people are not in touch or in tune with their body. Many people lose sensitivity to true stomach hunger, and get confused with multiple other emotional and physical signals. One of the first places to begin is with stomach hunger.

What is stomach hunger?

Stomach hunger, or physical hunger, actually involves a complex interaction between our digestive system or endocrine system and our brain. When the body feels hunger and needs refueling we start to feel weak and tired, sometimes finding it harder to concentrate and work. The stomach, which is located just below the rib cage, may start to ache and rumble. This is true stomach hunger and if we begin to eat in response to this we can feel our energy levels start to rise concentration levels start to become better because our body needs are being met.

I'm struggling...how do I know when to stop eating?

Hunger and fullness is regulated by the hypothalamus in the brain. When your body has had enough food to satisfy its needs, signals are sent to the hypothalamus. This is the part of the brain that registers our satiety. When we are in tune with our bodies we recognize that it's actually time to stop eating. Our stomach feels comfortable and satisfied, not stopped. We seem to begin to feel more alert, more energized and calmer.

It takes approximately 20 minutes for fullness signals to transmit from the stomach back to the brain. If you eat fast or you are not paying attention because you are either being distracted physically from your eating, like using a cell phone or television or because you are being distracted emotionally like numbing out or being in a guilt shame cycle you may not know when to stop eating. When you are distracted it's easy to override your fullness signals and eat much more than the body needs.

What can I do if I don't know when I am hungry and when I am full?

If you have been ignoring your hunger and fullness signals for a long time you may have temporarily lost your sensitivity to them. This can be the outcome of chronically restricting food intake, being raised to clean your plate, struggling with any kind of disordered eating, or using distractions emotionally or physically regularly while you are eating. If this is the case for you it will take some time to rediscover your hunger and fullness.

But all is not lost.

Many of my clients have learned and reconfigured their hunger and fullness signals with just a little bit of practice. One of the best ways to begin this process is to figure out which other ways you feel hunger.

You mean there are other ways to feel hunger?

Absolutely, but these are not necessarily physiological hunger! Hunger comes in many forms as we feel hunger both in our physical body and emotionally. These sensations are legitimate but they are not actual true stomach hunger. Here are some examples:

Teeth Hunger:

If you hold your stress, anxiety or worry in your jaw you may find that your teeth want to chew on something when you feel these emotions. In this instance our bodies are not calling for food, but we want to put things in our mouths to attempt to relieve our anxiety or stress.

Mouth Hunger:

This is the intense desire to taste a particular food. We may see, smell or think about something that we find so delicious our mouth starts to water. We can anticipate even tasting that food on our tongue. This, in fact, is not stomach hunger either.

Mind Hunger:

This is food that we have linked to specific times on the clock. It could be associated with specific meal or snack times. We may eat just because it is time even though we are not physically hungry.

Body Hunger:

When we feel certain emotions we hold those emotions particularly in specific parts of our body. It may be that when you are stressed you hunch your shoulders or squeeze your fists. In order to relieve the tension in our body we may choose food to relax.

Dehydration or Thirst:

It is easy to confuse the sluggishness of dehydration with actual hunger. The body may actually make you feel hungry as well if you are severely dehydrated as it receives water from the digestion and absorption process of food. However the body actually needs fluids, not food.

Tiredness:

When we are tired, we may sense that our energy levels are low. You may automatically think if you eat something, you'll feel better. Tiredness, however is NOT solved by food but by adequate rest and sleep patterns, something that is difficult for a lot of us.

Emotional Hunger:

This is a topic I will go into further in the next section of the book. However, in a nutshell, emotional hunger, is feeling emptiness emotionally due to an unmet emotional or spiritual need. Rather than acknowledge your feelings you try to fill the void with food. Or sometimes you may use food to stuff down your emotions so you do not feel anything at all. This is a process we call numbing and although there can be physical discomfort in the body it does not ever fill the need for the emotional discourse.

EMOTIONS AND EMOTIONAL EATING

Emotions are emotions, not emergencies.
--unknown

Many people do not recognize the role emotional eating plays in their health. Most blame a lack of willpower for the fact that 95% of all diets fail. Whether the diet fails from the start or when the dieter gains all the weight shortly after going off their diet, lack of willpower gets the blame. What many people don't realize is that emotional eating is often the real culprit. Research reports that up to 86% of dieters have some facets of emotional overeating. Not only does emotional eating play a pivotal role in weight gain and obesity, it also plays an important part in disorders such as anorexia, bulimia, and depression. In response to emotional stress people may overeat, binge on sugary, high fat snacks, reach for comfort foods or lose their appetite altogether. Weight goes up and down and this is all in an attempt to make yourself feel better—if only for the moment.

Emotional eating may be more difficult to address due to the complex interdependence with physiology.

There are 8 questions to ask yourself, to determine if you are an emotional overeater.

1. Do I eat when I am not hungry?
2. Do I sometimes eat much faster and/or much more than others?
3. Do I isolate form others so I can eat the way I want?
4. Do I sometimes think I will eat moderately and then eat much more than expected to eat?
5. Do I use food to numb out difficult feelings?
6. Can I over eat on almost any food?
7. Do I graze or snack frequently between meals?
8. Am I obsessive about the way I think about food?
9. Do I think that weight causes me serious physical and social problems and I still overeat?
10. Have I tried to stop bingeing and been unable to stay stopped?

If you answered yes to 2 or more of these questions, please read the rest of this section. It will be extremely helpful for you.

What can I do to stop giving in to my cravings?

First, right down which foods you crave making a list so you can see your craving patterns. For example look for things like tastes, textures and times of day. Some people crave sweet things while other people crave salty things, still others may crave anything with chocolate see what tastes you tend to crave most often. Is there a pattern to your craving? What is the pattern?

Times of day or night are also important because you can see if there is a pattern. Some people crave food because they let themselves get too hungry. If this is the case, this is a physiological craving. For physiological cravings you will need to add additional foods into your diet to help solve the issue.

Most of my clients respond to this suggestion with, "But I am trying to lose weight, I need to eat less not more" and in response, I say, "Yes but eating an extra apple and some nuts is a whole lot better for your body and weight loss then getting too hungry and eating a piece of cake."

So, for example, if you always crave specific foods in the afternoon you may want to increase your amount of food at lunch to see if it helps. More specifically increasing foods with fiber like fruits and vegetables are extremely helpful in helping you feel full longer.

Once you know your food-craving pattern, you can start to shift it by understanding it. As you breakdown the specific amount of the foods you crave you will know whether they soft and nurturing and comforting or whether they are hard and crunchy and provide a stress relief.

In our office I work with clients time and time again on this process in order to help them track, understand and reconfigure their patterns.

I will say it is definitely helpful to work with an outside, objective professional around these issues, if possible but I also recognize that clients can do some of this work on their own and become empowered in their own understanding of their eating.

Why do I over eat?

Overeating can be caused by a number of factors. First and foremost, I have seen individuals overeat when they under-eat earlier in the day. Including protein and fiber in all your meals and snacks is an excellent way to control hunger.

Fiber from foods such as fruits and vegetables act like a sponge to fill up your stomach. Protein stays in your stomach longer than either carbohydrates or fiber, keeping hunger at bay. Good sources of protein include seafood, nuts and lean meats. Make sure you include these satisfying foods at every meal to help keep you feeling full until the next meal.

Overeating can be the result of getting too tired as well. Make sure you keep your energy up by eating regularly and getting adequate rest, these things can make a world of difference with overeating patterns.

Emotional issues such as depression, loneliness, fear or anxiety can also cause overeating. In fact, a number of studies have linked depression and overeating in a direct causal relationship. This means that they are soft and nurturing or create each other and one can be linked to the other.

Understanding why you overeat is imperative in changing the behavior. Know why your overeating exists and the real reasons for your behavior.

Yes, you actually have REAL reasons or what I call "your intention" for overeating. Knowing this will create the change you need to change your overeating.

How do I stop?

There are a number of ways to stop the overeating cycle. In our clinic and my private practice I devise individualized solution options. The reasons behind overeating can be very complex and psychological in nature. However, in all my years in practice I have determined some general strategies that can provide amazing results.

First, make sure you are eating enough of protein, fiber and essential fatty acids throughout the day.

Second, if you do overeat make sure you put a small, balanced meal within three hours of the binge to enable blood sugar levels to stabilize.

One of the best strategies, however, is what I call the PAUSE.

Take a pause, When you feel like eating, pause for a moment and ask yourself, "Am I hungry?" Sometimes people get so focused on *what* they want to eat that they don't stop and ask themselves *why* they want to eat. If you use food as a coping tool, you may be out of touch with the cues that signal hunger or fullness, and it's important to bring your awareness back to your body.

I understand overeating and I know that people move fast before and sometimes during their overeating. Overeating is not a slow, mindful eating experience. So, first and foremost, SLOW DOWN, pause. Even if you have to set a timer for 60 seconds before you eat that food it helps to stop the quick compulsion to eat. Slowing down allows your brain to catch up to your body which can change how much or what you overeat.

How can I stop emotionally eating to lose weight? I eat when I am lonely, sad, happy or even excited.

You can and you are on the right track if this is an issue of yours.

First, you must understand your reasons for overeating. Figure out which of your emotions are linked to your overeating. Is it when you are sad, lonely, anxious, angry, frustrated or another emotion.

Then, think about what other things you can do besides eat when you feel that emotion. But, you must make sure the emotion matches the action. For example, don't try reading a book if you are angry; they don't match. If you're angry, go out for a walk, hike or throw a ball against a wall. Matching action and emotion is imperative.

If multiple emotions are linked to your overeating then it can be that you have not learned to tolerate feelings in general. This is true for a lot of emotional eaters. Know that you are not alone and you CAN change.

In our clinic, I work with clients specifically to match emotion to action so if this is difficult for you please remember you can seek an objective professional to help with this or contact our office for a referral or consult.

I keep trying to lose weight and change my eating but can't seem to stop eating sugar. I am a "Sugar Addict!" What do I do?

Well, aside from the increase in weight, diets high in sugar are strongly linked to an increased risk for type 2 diabetes, elevated triglycerides, low HDL (good) cholesterol levels, and heart disease. Sugar intake has also been linked to depression, migraines, poor eyesight, autoimmune diseases (such as arthritis, and multiple sclerosis), gout and osteoporosis. Even though everyone I speak to knows this it doesn't stop or change the behavior-in fact I think sometimes it even exacerbates it.

Recent research has shown that a high intake of carbohydrates, including sugar, releases a feel good chemical in the brain called serotonin. Think of how you feel after indulging in a high sugar meal or treat—almost euphoric, right? The high of a sugar rush is temporary though. After a few hours—or even a few minutes—you start to crash and you become tired, fatigued and lethargic. We also know that sugar coupled with various textures-like ooey, gooey foods increases dopamine in the brain.

Although sweet foods are tempting and delicious to most people (blame Mother Nature for that!), the more sugar you eat, the higher your tolerance becomes. So if you have a strong sweet tooth or intense cravings for sugar, chances are not that you were born that way, but that your dietary habits and food choices created the sugar monster you may have become.

Fortunately, we can reverse this tolerance in just a couple of weeks by cutting out sugar.

But that is not where we stop in this discussion because the truth is that "sugar addiction" is more complex. The other truth is that sugar has been around for centuries and "sugar addiction" has really only been spoken of in the last 50 years. In August 1492, Christopher Columbus stopped at La Gomera in the Canary Islands, for wine and water, intending to stay only four days. He became romantically involved with the governor of the island, Beatriz de Bobadilla y Ossorio, and stayed a month. When he finally sailed, she gave him cuttings of sugarcane, which became the first to reach the New World.

Today, we have so many other names and types of sugar it is difficult to identify all sources of sugar or even know if it is really the sugar which is tripping you up. Maybe it could be high fructose corn syrup? High fructose corn syrup, created in the 60's, one of the most addictive substances we know.

In order to cut back on hidden or added sugar, scan the ingredients list of a food label. If you see any of the following items listed, then sugar has been added to the product in one form or another and it is best left on the shelf at the store—especially if that sugar shows up within the first five ingredients of any food product.

Agave nectar	Corn syrup solids	Grape juice concentrate
Agave syrup	Crystallized fructose	Honey
Barley malt	Date sugar	Invert sugar
Beet sugar	Dextran	Lactose
Brown rice syrup	Dextrose	Malt
Brown sugar	Yellow Sugar	Maltodextrin
Buttered syrup	Diastatic malt	Maltose
Cane sugar	Evaporated cane juice	Maple syrup
Cane juice	Fructose	Molasses
Cane juice crystals	Fruit juice	Raw sugar
Carob syrup	Fruit juice concentrate	Refiner's syrup
Confectioner's sugar	Glucose	Sorghum syrup
Corn syrup	Glucose solids	Sucanat
High fructose corn syrup	Golden sugar	Sucrose
Corn sugar	Golden syrup	Sugar
Corn sweetener	Grape sugar	Turbinado sugar

I have had so many clients in the past label themselves as a "sugar addict" and my first question always is, "Are you really a sugar addict or do you really just believe you are a sugar addict?" In order to understand more about yourself and your relationship to sugar, you must do 4 things.

1. Identify if sugar is the issue or if it is one of the other ingredients listed above?

2. Are non-nutritive sweeteners part of the problem?-

3. Is it a physical thing or psychological? Are you eating enough healthful, nutritious food with adequate fiber and protein during the day? Or is it truly a brain chemistry piece?

   I have had many clients come to me thinking they were addicted to sugar only to realize they were actually undernourished with specific nutrients thus leading to excess sugar and carbohydrate cravings. It is extremely important to recognize if you have a deficiency of a macro or micro nutrient leading to sugar cravings.

4. Is it a belief or identity construct, engrained? What you say to yourself is what you believe. It is imperative you know what you are saying to yourself about yourself. It is these things that shape what we do. Our beliefs determine our actions, thoughts, emotions and behaviors. In believing you are a sugar addict, you will behave like a sugar addict.

Beliefs construct the silent GPS that covertly dictates the course of our eating and our life.

Know that true "sugar addiction" is very controversial. You may have an emotional connection to foods that contain sugar, you may have a physical deprivation instigating sugar cravings or you may have a nutritional deficit initiating sugar cravings to quell the deficiency. True sugar addiction is complex and actually is not complex

Understanding specific kinds of sugary foods you crave can help you identify other clues to this eating pattern for you. Is it chocolate, ice cream, cookies, cakes etc? Be specific, it is important to gain clarity about the specific types of foods and quantities with which you have difficulty. Get a sense of the tastes and textures these foods have. Are they smooth and creamy or sweet and crunchy? The texture of foods combined with the flavors can definitely be a component of the "addiction."

Identifying and understanding the exact nature of all of these specific factors that surround your sugar intake can lead to ultimate freedom and empowerment. You can then take action around what may or may not be your sugar addiction but before you succeed you must know what you actually believe and what your body beholds in its infinite wisdom.

Does stress really effect weight gain?

Absolutely! Stress releases cortisol, which increases your body's ability to store fat particularly around your midsection. Stress can also increase your cravings for certain foods and the quantities of foods you may eat. Creating a stress management component of your weight loss program is essential for long-term sustainability.

I heard the amount of sleep you get can actually effect your weight loss. Is this true?

Absolutely true as well! Irregular sleep patterns can create cortisol issues, which can increase our bodies fat storage ability as mentioned above. Furthermore, sleep is actually when our healing processes occur. This is when your body dumps toxins into the lymphatic system processing them for excretion. Without proper sleep proper detoxification, healing and repair cannot occur.

Sleep is also when your body replenishes itself and all of its various hormones, such as insulin, cortisol, thyroid stimulating hormone and reproductive hormones and all which have been mentioned previously in questions answered in this book.

Let's not forget how sleep is important for brain and body function. You will function and feel much better with a good night sleep then you will without. Counting those sheep is essential for energy levels and metabolism.

I eat at night, sometimes even waking up at night to eat. What can I do?

Night eating is a more common behavior than many people or practitioners realize. There is so much shame for my clients in this area. In fact, after speaking with so many clients over the last 20 plus years, I would actually say this is the most underreported and undertreated symptom my clients have had.

There are two different facets of night eating. Some of you may eat throughout the night prior to bedtime, filling an emotional hunger or one that may exist from physical hunger itself. You see, if you do not eat enough during the day, you will eat more during the evening. I have had so many clients that feel like they have "done good" on their diet, only to be starving when they get home at night and overeat throughout the night to fill the hunger that exists from the under consumption during the day. The problem is that emotions and tiredness are more intense in the evening and so overeating can become inevitable.

The second type of night eating is more complex psychologically and happens right before bedtime and/or throughout the evening as someone wakes up from sleep. As taken from Wikipedia, **night eating syndrome (NES)** is an eating disorder, characterized by a delayed circadian pattern of food intake. Research diagnostic criteria have been proposed[1] and include evening hyperphagia (consumption of 25% or more of the total daily calories after the evening meal) and/or nocturnal awakening and ingestion of food two or more times per week. The person must have awareness of the night eating to differentiate it from the parasomnia sleep-related eating disorder (SRED). Three of five associated symptoms must also be present: lack of appetite in the morning, urges to eat in the evening/at night, belief that one must eat in order to fall back to sleep at night, depressed mood, and/or difficulty sleeping. NES affects both men and women, between 1 and 2% of the general population, and approximately 10% of obese individuals.

If you struggle with night eating, there is help. But in this arena as with all diagnostic eating disorders or disordered eating patterns I do recommend getting professional help from a specialist like myself who is familiar and excellent in their treatment philosophy and approach to help you identify, understand and change these behavioral, psychological and emotional patterns.

You mentioned tracking and understanding my patterns with my emotions and eating. How can I understand my emotions and my eating better?

First and foremost find a tool that can help you objectively understand your patterns better. In our clinic and with our clients I use a Food Emotion Tracker (FET) to help them understand their patterns better. However, there are many variations of food journals on line. Find one that works for you and helps you track and understand your patterns better.

Second, get reflective, objective help. This can be in the format of group support, individual therapeutic treatment or self paced learning. I developed an on-line, 8 module course with audio, video and workbook content for people with overeating issues to target your cognitive understanding of your overeating. This can be found at www.EmpowermentCoachingInternational.com under the courses section. In our clinic, we also offer weekly group calls for our community to enable them to learn new content about various facets of eating, behavior, emotion and life and provide a safe sounding board for questions and help in an anonymous format.

"Knowing the change and doing the change are only separated by action"-anonymous

Food Emotion Tracker (FET)

Date: _____ Mon Tues Wed Thurs Fri Sat Sun Water Intake: ___oz.

Time	Types of Food You Are Eating	Reason for Eating	Appetite and Cravings	Feelings Before and After Eating	Portion Size	Who Were You with?	Did You Eat Hurriedly or Calmly?	Were You Doing Another Activity While Eating?
11 am	Potato chips	Bored	Salt Craving	None/Content	2 Handfuls	Husband	Hurriedly	Watching TV

What's Your Mood: *exhausted, angry, sad, frustrated, stressed, depressed, overwhelmed, anxious, lonely, jealous, bored, hopeful, content, happy, thrilled, etc.*

Objective Reflection on the Day:_____

_____

_____

Patterns I want to Change and Solutions:_____

_____

_____

Patient Success Story
Meet Jamie C.

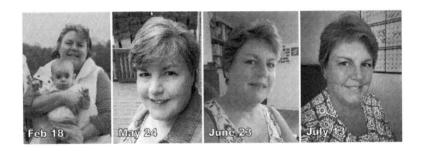

I've spent all of my adult life battling my weight and yo-yo dieting. I am one of 5 girls. Three of my sisters have been diagnosed with cancer (2 with breast, 1 with cervical). Only one is a survivor. When my father passed away from Alzheimer's in December 2015 and then my baby sister in April 2016 I became depressed. From December 2016 to the Anniversary of my youngest sister's death depression got really bad. And I would seek out sugar to try and make myself feel better.

Watching Dr. Francis' ads I realized that something had to change. I could not continue on the path I was taking. When I met with Dr. Francis, his question to me was "Why now?" My reply, "Three of my sisters have had cancer and two did not survive, if I am going to get cancer it was not going to be because I didn't try to prevent it."

I have dieted all of my life (going to WW for the first time when I was middle school age) and would lose 20 lbs. >\< time and again. I would hit a plateau and give up only to gain it all back and some. With Dr. Francis' program change was almost immediate. Cravings are gone. It sounds cliché but the truth is I have not felt this good since before my children were born (they are 27 and 24). The first thing people notice about me is not my weight loss but my complexion. They tell me I am glowing. I am full of energy. My blood pressure is no longer an issue. My joints no longer ache. I really am glowing. I find myself smiling so much more these days.

Feeling Amazing! - Jamie C.

SOME SCRUMPTIOUS RECIPES FOR YOUR SUCCESS

EATING HEALTHFULLY CAN BE TASTY TOO!

5 Quick and Easy Recipes

HEALTHY CHICKEN PICCATA

INGREDIENTS:

3 ounces skinless, boneless chicken breasts, cut in half
1 teaspoon coconut oil
¼ teaspoon Himalayan sea salt
¼ teaspoon pepper
½ cup chicken broth, low sodium
2 garlic cloves, minced
1 lemon, thinly sliced
1 tablespoon fresh parsley, chopped

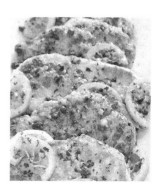

INSTRUCTIONS:

1. Place each chicken breast portion between two pieces of plastic wrap. Using the flat side of a meat mallet, pound each breast until it's about ¼ inch thick.
2. Remove top plastic wrap and salt and pepper chicken.

3. Add coconut oil to a large sauté pan and lay chicken salted side down, then salt and pepper this side of chicken.
4. Cook chicken until browned and no longer pick in center, turning halfway through cooking. Remove chicken and set aside in a covered container to keep warm.
5. Add garlic to hot sauté pan and cook for about a minute or until browned. Add chicken broth and scrap any brown bits from the sauté pan, bring to a boil.
6. Add lemon slices, cover and reduce to low heat.
7. Cook until lemon slices are softened about 4-5 minutes.
8. Return chicken to pan and heat through.
9. Serve chicken with lemon juices over top and sprinkle with parsley.

TACO STUFFED ZUCCHINI BOATS

INGREDIENTS:

1 medium zucchini
1 teaspoon extra virgin olive oil
2 cloves garlic
3 ounces ground turkey
½ teaspoon chili powder
½ teaspoon onion powder
¼ teaspoon garlic powder
¼ teaspoon oregano
1 teaspoon cumin
1 teaspoon smoked paprika
¼ teaspoon Himalayan Sea Salt
1 ½ cups diced cherry tomatoes
Optional topping: Cilantro, 1/8 avocado, shredded lettuce

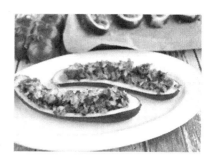

INSTRUCTIONS:

1. Preheat the oven to 400 degrees Fahrenheit.
2. Scoop out the insides of the zucchini with a spoon or melon scooper and chop them.
3. Add the chopped zucchini to a large skillet.
4. Place the scooped out zucchini shells into a 9 by 13 baking dish. (If you prefer a softer zucchini, place this dish in the oven and cook for about 15 minutes then scoop the cooked filling into the zucchini boats and bake as directed below).

5. Cook the chopped zucchini with extra virgin olive oil and garlic on medium heat and add the turkey.
6. Once the turkey is browned, add the seasonings, and cherry tomatoes. Continue to cook for a few more minutes.
7. Fill zucchini with this mixture.
8. Cover and bake 20-25 minutes or until zucchini is tender.
9. Enjoy with cilantro, shredded lettuce and 1/8 avocado!

ANTIPASTO CAULIFLOWER RICE SALAD

INGREDIENTS:

2 heads cauliflower or 8 cups florets
1 tablespoon extra-virgin olive oil
6 ounces artichokes in the jar, sliced
6 ounces roasted red peppers, chopped
6 pitted olives, sliced
1 cup fresh basil, chopped
3 tablespoons apple cider vinegar
Himalayan sea salt and pepper, to taste

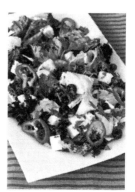

INSTRUCTIONS:

1. Preheat oven to 400 degrees Fahrenheit.
2. Place cauliflower florets on two baking pans.
3. Toss florets with extra virgin olive oil.
4. Bake for 1 hour or until tender.
5. Place cooked florets into a food processor and pulse until texture of rice.
6. Pour into a large serving bowl and allow to cool.
7. Once cooled add remaining ingredients into bowl and toss together.
8. Taste and adjust Himalayan sea salt and pepper to your preference.
9. Serve room temperature immediately or keep refrigerated until ready to serve.

RED CABBAGE COLESLAW

INGREDIENTS:

6 cups (about ½ head) shredded red cabbage
6 tablespoons lemon juice
¼ cup apple cider vinegar
¼ cup extra virgin olive oil
2 teaspoons dried basil
1 clove garlic (minced)
1 stalk celery (minced)
1 cup watermelon (diced)
Himalayan sea salt and pepper, to taste

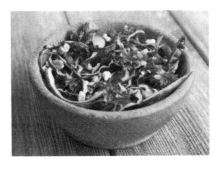

INSTRUCTIONS:

1. Shred the cabbage and set aside.
2. In a large mixing bowl, whisk the lemon, extra virgin olive oil, and vinegar. Stir in the basil, garlic and celery. Place the shredded cabbage into the dressing and toss to combine.
3. Top with diced watermelon and Himalayan sea salt and pepper. Toss gently.
4. For best results, let coleslaw chill a few hours before serving.

VEGETABLE PESTO EGG SKILLET

INGREDIENTS:

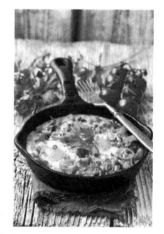

Pesto: (Serving Size = 1 teaspoon)
1 cup fresh basil
1 cup fresh kale
1/3 cup raw slivered almonds or
regular almonds
2 large cloves garlic
1 teaspoon lemon juice
1 teaspoon Himalayan sea salt
½ teaspoon freshly ground pepper
Optional: ¼ teaspoon red pepper flakes
2 tablespoons extra-virgin olive oil

EVERYTHING ELSE:

1 teaspoon grass-fed butter
2 cups vegetables of your choice
2 whole eggs

INSTRUCTIONS:

1. Heat butter in a skillet
2. Add in sliced vegetables and let cook for 5 minutes
3. Add in 1 tablespoon of water and cover skillet with a lid
4. After 5 minutes, remove lid and toss vegetables
5. While cooking a little while longer, toss pesto ingredients into your high-speed blender

6. Pour 1 teaspoon pesto over vegetables and toss until fully coated
7. Crack in eggs and let cook for 5-10 minutes (I cover mine for 3-4 minutes in the middle)
8. Once egg whites are opaque, remove from heat, sprinkle with red pepper flakes and serve hot

CAULIFLOWER FRIED RICE

INGREDIENTS:

1 cup cauliflower, grated
1 cup onion, chopped
1 cup zucchini, chopped
1 cup broccoli, grated
1 cup spinach, finely chopped
2 teaspoons extra virgin olive oil
4 cloves garlic, crushed
¼ cup scallions, chopped
2 organiceggs1 1tablespoon garlic powder
1 teaspoon onion powder
½ teaspoon red pepper flakes (more to taste)
1-2 tablespoons Bragg's Liquid Aminos, more to taste
½ teaspoon Himalayan sea salt, more to taste
½ teaspoon freshly ground pepper

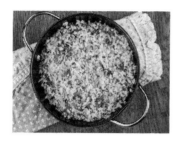

INSTRUCTIONS:

1. Using your food processor or cheese grater, pulse/grate cauliflower until rice consistency
2. Cut up all veggies you're going to use and set aside
3. In one pan, heat 1 teaspoon extra virgin olive oil and sauté 2 cloves crushed garlic, add in onions and sauté for 5 minutes, then add in the rest of your veggies (except for spinach) and mix well for 6-8 minutes

4. Add cauliflower rice to the pan and mix well, let cook for 5 minutes, stirring often.
5. Make a hole in the center of your rice and put eggs in. Once scrambled in the center, mix in completely with the rice. Add scallions and mix again.
6. Add garlic powder, onion powder, red pepper flakes, Himalayan sea salt and pepper, and Bragg's Liquid Aminos and mix well.
7. Add spinach and mix until sautéed.
8. Taste and adjust spices as desired.

CONCLUSION

In this book we have answered many different questions about weight loss surrounding the physical, physiological and psychological aspects of change. These provide different essential keys to both weight loss and sustainable weight management.

The first thing you want to do is take action on what you have discovered in these chapters. When changing anything in life you must know that taking action is the key to success.

Just take one step at a time. I know lots of people come to our office looking for a magic bullet but doing the things that we mentioned in the book and correcting these problems will allow you to have rapid success.

It all boils down to becoming your own health advocate and having not only an understanding of what you do and why do it but having the distinctions and energy to move through and make that change. Your health is your number one asset in life. As my grandfather used to say, "If you have your health you have everything."

The great part about it is you have control of your health every second of every day when you wake up from dusk until dawn.

Understanding the information we talked about in these chapters will allow you to understand how to create long-lasting change for yourself. Enabling you to uncover your best you through various facets of physical, physiological and psychological change.

Our hope in writing this book is that this information will help you with the changes you need to make, but if you cannot lose at least 3 pounds per week on your own, or are taking medications that are hindering you from weight change, or are over the age of 40 and have metabolic or emotional issues please email us at askdrfrancis@gmail.com and set up a free consultation with us.

Once we start you on your program, you will finally be able to take massive action and see tremendous results with your weight loss and all your health goals. During our office visit you will have an individual appointment with one of us or one of our team specialists. You can find us at www.DrCharlesFrancis.com and can fill out the paperwork found on this website.

That will provide us the information we need to make all the recommendations that will help you with your success. This visit should take no more than 45 minutes. These 45 minutes will make you healthier than you were 4 to 5 years ago. Allowing you to reach a new level of energy, health, and confidence moving forward in your life.

Once you have emailed us, one of our clinical team members will contact you directly to set up your free, life-changing appointment today. Isn't it time YOU put YOU first?

We are looking forward to helping you achieve all of your success.